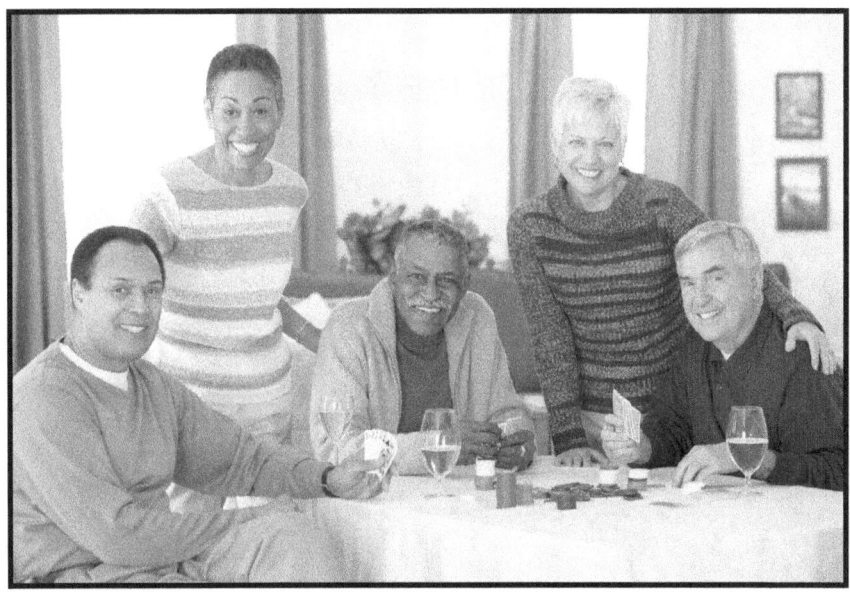

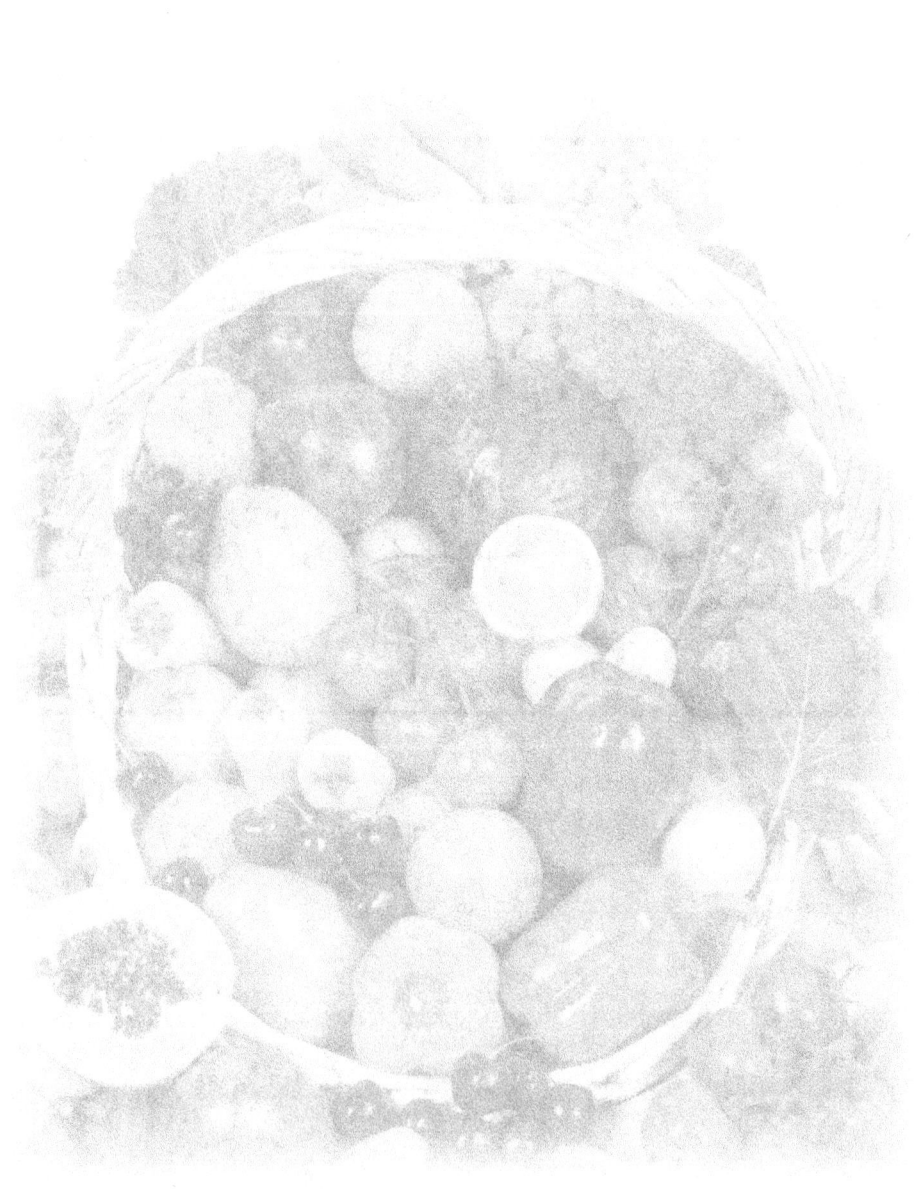

Recipes and Meal Planning for the Happy Healthy Senior

Seniors Can Eat Happy, and Healthy

by

Diana Darrisaw

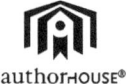

authorHOUSE®

AuthorHouse™
1663 Liberty Drive, Suite 200
Bloomington, IN 47403
www.authorhouse.com
Phone: 1-800-839-8640

First published by AuthorHouse 8/14/2008

ISBN: 978-1-4343-7652-7 (sc)

Printed in the United States of America
Bloomington, Indiana

This book is printed on acid-free paper.

My name is Diana Darrisaw. I am a retired patient care food supervisor. I was a member of DMA, the Dietary Managers Association, for more than twenty years. I have national certification for supervision in patient care. I had membership in HFSS, the Hospital Food Service Society for more than ten years. Working with menu-planning with seniors for thirty-five years in the top hospitals in the Philadelphia area was the best degree I ever could have earned.

It gave me pleasure and comfort in writing Recipe and Meal Planning. Since I am a senior with certain food allowances, I recognize eating can be a problem. Certain illnesses do connect with foods. We as the elderly share a very special connection I call Seniorhood. This is our time to have every thing that is special and our health is number one. Proper eating will encourage a healthier you. As I share my thoughts and beliefs with other seniors, I have found we have quite a bit in common concerning our food restrictions. Showing you the menus that have been a part of my meals hopefully will encourage you that healthy eating can be happy. By using removal and replacement in meal-planning, I adapted ways and means in making mealtime great for those with conditions like high blood pressure, cardiac disorder, and diabetes. In using the recipes I have shared, hopefully your menu planning will offer you healthier and happier meals. In my first book; (Happy, Healthy, Seniors) I wanted to give the reader motivation, and education. The beginner needs to understand that you can change to a new way of food preparation and cooking. This book goes a step further but in the same direction to obtain better health.

The ingredients used are available in any average supermarket. The recipes shared are low in cost, salt, sugar, fats, and cholesterol. The best part is this: FLAVOR will return to your mouth again! Sweet and savory will be back in your life without fearing your next appointment with the doctor! I can share the recipes, but the rest is up to you. We all know our boundaries to keep good health. If you have restrictions in your choices of foods, this is the helper you need in your kitchen. Always check with your physician before any change in diet.

REVIEW

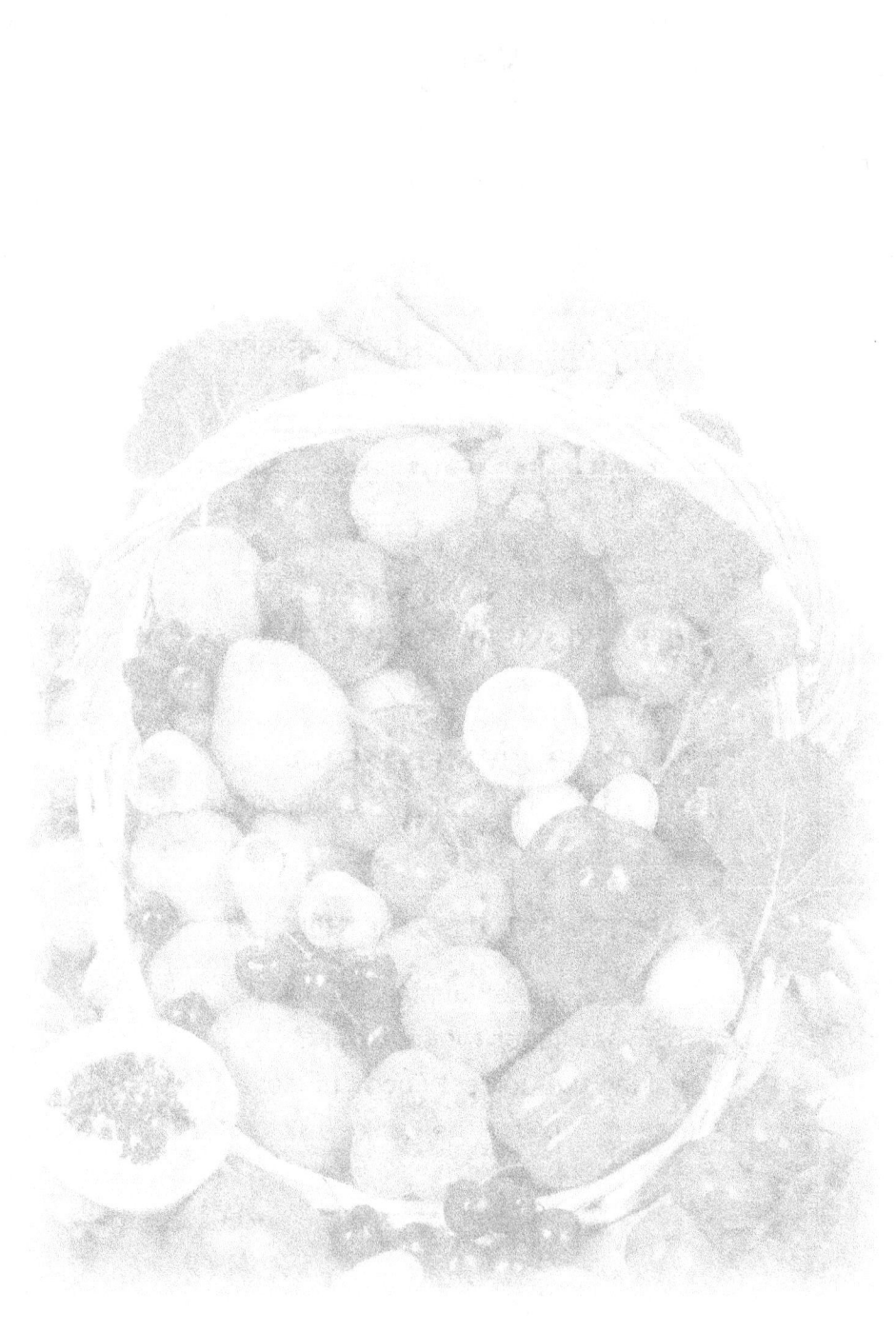

CHAPTER ONE

MEAT THE BEST IT CAN BE

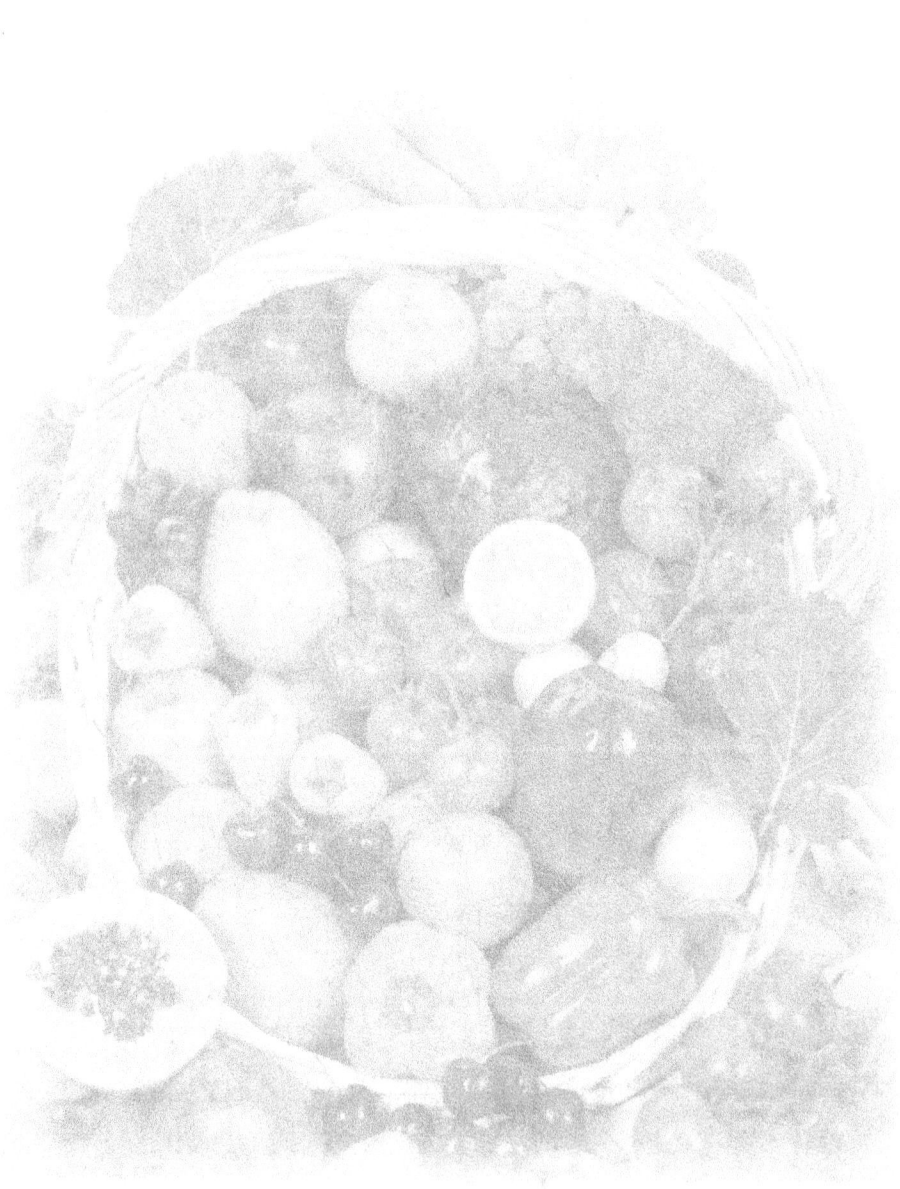

Spicy Miniature Meat Loaves
Yield 2 servings

½ lb. ground beef

½ lb. ground turkey

1 medium chopped onion

1 mild chopped chili pepper

1 tbsp. fresh parsley

1 level tbsp. garlic powder

1 egg white

2 tbsp. ketchup

2 tbsp. plain bread crumbs

Cook onion and, cleaned chili pepper in a non-stick skillet under medium heat. When tender add to uncooked meat in a large bowl. Combine dry ingredients, your favorite low sodium seasoning, one beaten egg white, and ketchup. Divide mixture into two portions, and mold into loaves. Bake in preheated oven at 350 degrees for 20 to 25 minutes.

Ground beef is simple and fast to cook, but the fat and calories can be high. Using a lean beef or ground turkey can cut down on fat and calories. I prefer a 50/50 mixture. I also recommend seasoning with **Chef Paul's Magic Salt-free Seasoning** You don't miss the salt at all. Don't forget to wash your hands well after handling chilies.

Quick Chili
Yield 2 to 3 servings

2 lbs. ground turkey
1½ cups vegetarian baked beans
1 small chopped onion
1 small mild chopped chili
½ cup shredded smoked cheddar, low-salt and
    -cholesterol cheese

Bring out the nonstick skillet and spray lightly with a plain cooking spray. Add ground meat, and onions, chili (open and clean chili out well, remove seeds and white veins). Wash hands!

When turkey and other ingredients are done, add beans and bean juice. Stir well, heating on stove over low heat until all ingredients are completely hot. Add cheese just before serving.

Chilies are packed with vitamins A and C, and offer other good nutrition.

Always drain excess fats from meats.
Make a nonstick skillet and saucepan a part of your cooking equipment. It can reduce the amount of fat needed.

Skinless Chicken with Peaches

2-3 oz. portions of uncooked chicken
(any type of chicken will be fine)
2 tbsp. unsalted margarine
15oz can of unsweetened sliced peaches
1 chopped onion
herbal cooking spray
½ cup chicken broth

Wash chicken well, and remove skin. Season chicken with low sodium seasoning, and spray medium preheated skillet; add chicken, onions and broth.

Cook for 30 minutes covered until done. Add peach slices, juice, and margarine to skillet after chicken has completely cooked. Baste chicken well with pan juices. Serve sliced peaches along with chicken.

Buffalo Stew
Yield 3 servings

2 lb. buffalo cubes

4 cups water (water should cover all the
   ingredients)

2 cups cooked brown rice

½ cup peas (frozen)

1 cup carrots (frozen)

1 bay leaf

2 stalks of chopped fresh celery

1 large diced onion

cornstarch

all-purpose unsalted seasonings

Cover meat with water, season to taste, add celery, onions, bay leaf. Cook on top stove in large skillet with lid on medium heat until meat is tender and fully cooked. Stir in cornstarch. One teaspoon of cornstarch in four ounces of water, stir until cornstarch has dissolved, add to cooking skillet slowly to make gravy. Add rice, peas, and carrots. Lower heat and cook for 10 minutes covered.

Buffalo is lean, tasty, a new meat for most, full of good flavor. It has a taste very similar to beef. Cornstarch is a great choice for thickening. Remember to remove bay leaf when pot is done.

Turkey Pasta Melt
Yield 2 to 3 servings

2 lbs. ground turkey

1½ cups of elbow pasta

2 crushed garlic cloves

1 small cleaned green pepper, diced

4 oz. tomato sauce

16 oz. crushed tomatoes

½ cup ricotta cheese

½ cup shredded parmesan cheese

Brown ground turkey, onions, peppers, and garlic. Add to meat, tomato sauce and crushed tomatoes. Add cooked pasta and cheeses. Blend and season together well. Reduce heat to low until cheese has melted.

Why turn on the oven if not necessary? Casserole dishes can be cooked and finished on a top burner.

A pinch of sugar can lower the acid in tomato dishes.

Creamed Chipped Chicken
Yield 2 servings

4 portions of minute chicken steak
  (used for Philly cheese steak)
½ cup chopped onions (onions are always
  optional)
 ½ cup red bell peppers, diced
¼ tsp. chicken base (low salt)
12 oz. low-fat milk
Melba back toast, or regular toast

In a nonstick pan, cook chicken steak, onions, and peppers over medium heat until browned.

In a saucepan, heat 10 oz. of the milk over medium heat; when hot, add chicken base, and thicken with a flour and milk paste (1 tbsp. of flour, mixed with 2 oz. of the remaining milk). Blend together until smooth. Add to cooking milk, stir until thickened. Add chicken mixture. Stir well, remove from heat.

How many times have we eaten creamed chipped beef? This is a new turn for creamed meat.
1 tbsp. flour will not tumble your diet.

Chicken base is a dry ingredient that adds extra flavor.

Sauerkraut Steamed Pork Loin Chops
Yield 3 servings

3 cups canned sauerkraut (drained)

3 large lean pork loin chops, or 4 small

¼ tsp. black pepper

2 medium cored and peeled, Granny Smith
    apples, (diced small)

1 medium diced onion

3 tbsp. dry parsley

(no salt needed)

In a nonstick preheated skillet place washed and seasoned loin chops with onions. Cook covered over medium heat for 15 minutes. Remove lid and add sauerkraut and diced apples. Return lid and cook for 30 minutes until apples are fork tender. Garnish with parsley

Sauerkraut is ready to eat when purchased. The sodium can be high, so rinse under cool water for 5 minutes before using to dissolve some of the salty juices. This style of cabbage in the can offers good calcium and has vitamin C also.

Buy the loin of fresh pork; it offers a lot of good nutrition and less fat.

Chicken with Tomato Basil Rice
Yield 3 servings

6 oz. skinless chicken breast

3 cups cooked rice (your choice)

2 tbsp. unsalted margarine

2 cups tomato sauce

2 chopped garlic cloves, or 1 tbsp. garlic
   powder

1 tbsp. ground basil

Wash skinless chicken well and cut in bite size portions. Season the chicken with basil, garlic powder, and all-purpose unsalted seasonings. Place in a preheated nonstick skillet, sprayed with olive oil cooking spray. Cook chicken over medium heat for 10 minutes   Add cooked rice, margarine, and crushed tomatoes; cover and heat for 20 minutes.

Since chicken is so popular, the more recipes we can share the better eating for all.

Three oz. of chicken breast can be slightly high in calories, but the vitamin B3 (niacin) is fabulously high. B6 and phosphorus are showing their heads also. This is a good source of protein. Keep the skin off when eating chicken. It is important to cook chicken thoroughly. Salmonella is still on the rise.

Beef Jubilee
Yield 2 to 3 servings

2 lbs. lean beef cubes

2 large celery stalks, chopped

2 cups cooked elbow macaroni

1 large diced onion

10 oz. box frozen cauliflower

10 oz. box frozen French cut green beans

2 tbsp. sour cream

3 cups low sodium beef broth

1 cup water

2 tbsp. unsalted margarine

2 tsp. all-purpose flour

Wash beef well, and place in a pot with 3 cups beef broth and 1 cup water.

Cook over medium heat. Add onions, celery, margarine, seasonings, and let cook for 20minutes. Take flour and mix with 4 ounces of water. Stir mixture into the pot. Lower heat, add thawed, drained vegetables. Let simmer for one hour. Add pasta and take off heat. Garnish with sour cream when serving.

Beef is a good source of protein, selenium, vitamin B12, and much more. Frozen vegetables are minutes away from being ready to eat when purchased.

Beef Potato Pancakes

2 cups cooked mashed seasoned potatoes
2 oz. cooked chopped beef
Low sodium seasonings
2 tbsp. egg substitute
2 chopped fine scallion bulbs (no stems)
Cooking spray

Preheat and lightly spray skillet. In a bowl, mix potatoes, beef, seasonings, onions, eggs. Blend well, make hand patties. (Use an ice-cream dipper, remove from dipper, round off, and flatten.) The size is your choice. This is a recipe for two to three patties. Brown over medium heat, uncovered.

Plain baked medium skin on potato offer vitamin B6, copper, potassium, vitamin C, low sodium and calories are high. Cut down on a low nutrient but high calorie food in order to enjoy a potato.

Leftover potatoes are perfect for this recipe.

Mint and Cranberry-flavored Lamb Chops
Yield 2 servings

4 lean lamb chops (small choices)
1½ tbsp. crushed mint
2 -1 inch slices unsweetened cranberry sauce
½ tsp. rosemary
½ tsp. black pepper
Butter flavored cooking spray
2 tbsp. goat cheese

Wash meat well; trim extra fat. Rub with a mixture of rosemary, mint, and pepper.

Cook in a medium-sized, sprayed skillet. Cook covered, turn meat until done. Turn off heat, garnish lamb with goat cheese, and cover. Serve with cranberry sauce.

Lamb is a meat that many people have not adapted a taste for. Mint and rosemary are good partners for lamb.

Veal Italia

3 veal chops

6 oz. of your favorite spaghetti sauce

Oregano

Basil to taste

1 cup diced tomato

2 cups cooked penne pasta

1 medium diced onion

½ cup red and green peppers

2 chopped garlic cloves

10 oz. box chopped frozen drained spinach

1 tsp. black pepper

1 tsp. onion powder

2 tbsp. feta cheese

Heat large nonstick skillet. Season chops with dry seasoning. Begin to brown chops. Add onions, peppers, and chopped garlic; when tender, add tomato, sauce, and cooked spinach. Make sure spinach is drained or dried off. Cover and cook over low heat for 30 minutes. Remove lid and add cooked pasta. Add more garlic or olive oil to desired taste. When ready to serve, garnish with feta cheese.

Veal is another source of protein that people are eating more of.

CHAPTER ONE A

MEAT SUBSTITUTES DISHES

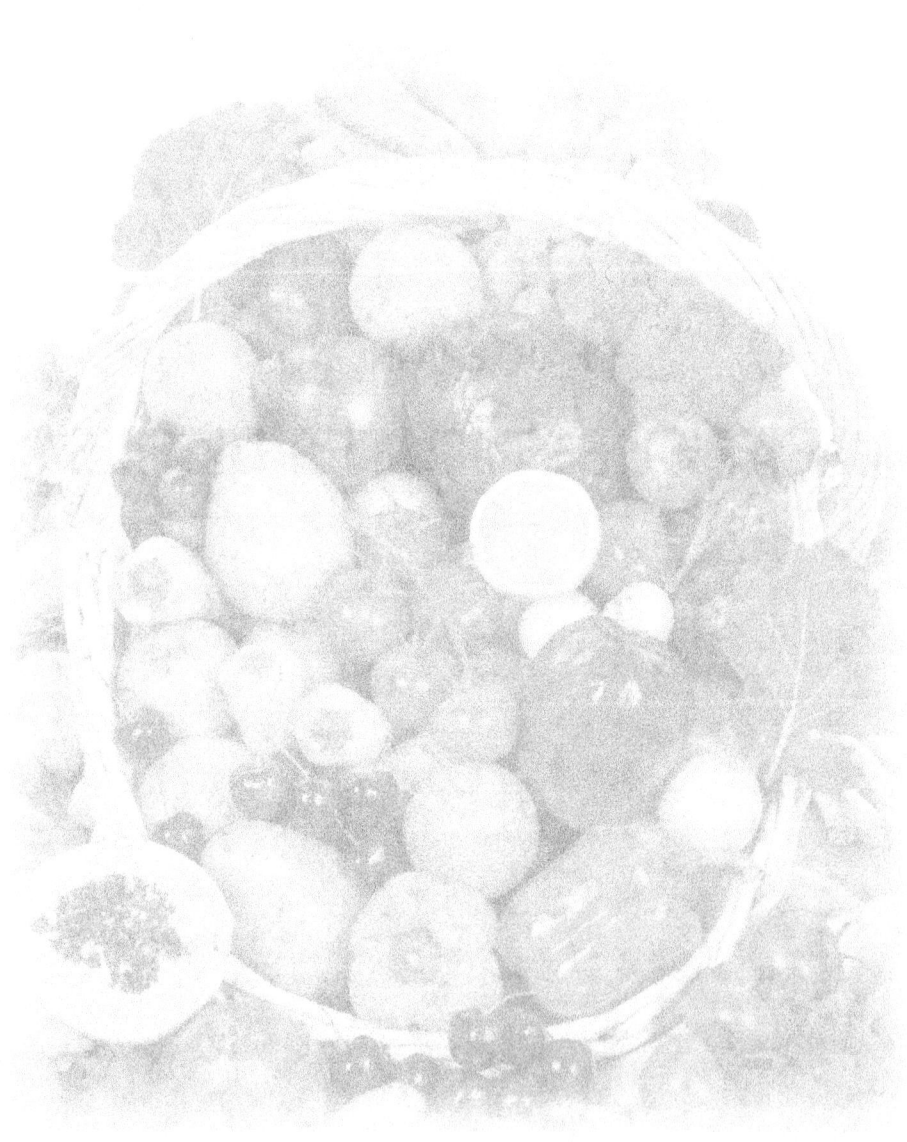

Corn and Cheese Pudding
Yield 3 to 4 servings

1 cup creamed corn

1 cup whole-kernel corn

2½ tbsp. unsalted margarine

2 egg whites

2 cups low-fat creamy cottage cheese

½ cup low-fat milk

¼ tsp. black pepper

¼ cup chopped parsley

Drain whole-kernel corn; add both corns to a bowl. Add melted margarine, pepper, parsley, beaten egg whites, milk, and cottage cheese. Mix all ingredients together, and place in a casserole dish. Cook in a preheated 250-degree oven for 10 to 15 minutes.

Garnish with parsley.

Yellow fresh kernel corn contains two important antioxidants: Lutein and Zeaxanthin. These are great for the eyes.

A FLUFF AND BUFF High-protein Omelet

I named this after my cats, Fluff and Buff. They love eggs!

Yield 2 servings

1 cup egg substitute

½ cup shredded low-fat cheese (skim mild jack cheese)

¼ cup cooked green peas

1 small chopped mild onion

2 tbsp. low-fat milk

Spray nonstick skillet with butter-flavored cooking spray. Place over medium heat.

While skillet is heating, assemble ingredients together.

In a medium bowl, beat together eggs and milk. Add onions, peas, and cheese; stir all ingredients together. Pour into skillet. As the edges begin to firm, gently fold in half in pan.

Green peas offer protein. If you have been told to lay off the eggs every day, replace that regular egg with egg whites or egg substitute.

Soy Cheese Sandwich (2 sandwiches)

6 oz. sliced soy cheese

4 slices whole-grain bread

½ cup romaine lettuce

½ cup shredded carrots

¼ cup sliced red onion

¼ cup thin-sliced yellow peppers

1 tsp light mayonnaise

1 tsp mild mustard

Mix mustard and mayonnaise together before applying on the bread. Add two slices of cheese to each sandwich.

Place lettuce, carrots, onion, and peppers. Place the tops on and you have your sandwich. You have proteins, fats, and carbohydrates.

Try some tofu, soy milk, and beans. It could be a new healthy, happy step.

Fruit and Cottage Cheese Plate
Yield 2 servings

2 cup creamy low-fat cottage cheese

Leafy mixed red and green lettuce

½ cup sliced fresh strawberries

½ cup sliced unsweetened canned peaches

½ cup sliced unsweetened pineapple

¼ cup mandarin oranges

8 oz. vanilla yogurt

Place cheese on a large platter with a bed of mixed lettuce.

Don't remove the tops of the strawberries until ready to slice. Place on lettuce, with drained peaches and pineapples, and mandarin oranges. Top with your favorite yogurt.

If you remove the green door on your strawberries, the vitamin C starts running away.

Cottage cheese is a good meat substitute. Keep the fat low.

Tofu Happy Blend
Yield 2 to 3 servings

6 oz. of firm tofu, cubed

½ cup beef stock or broth

½ cup chicken stock or broth

¼ tsp. black pepper

1 large onion cut in thin rings

1 cup julienne sliced yellow squash

1 medium red bell pepper, seeded and cut
   julienne

Assemble all vegetables the day before; place in water and chill well.

Place 2 oz. of tofu in the beef broth, and 2 oz. in the chicken broth; make sure all the content is covered with the broths for 2hrs. Put tofu into strainer to drain excess liquid over-night in refrigerator. When ready to cook, bring out a large skillet, spray well using an olive oil or garlic-flavored cooking spray. Place over medium high heat. While skillet is heating, drain vegetables. Mix tofu and stir fry for 5minutes. Add all of vegetables to skillet. Takes about 5 minutes to cook.

Keep the skin on as many vegetables as possible when cook-ing. Tofu is popular as a meat substitute for the young at heart. Tofu is a great flavor-grabber.

Vegetable-stuffed Fish
Yield 2 to 3 servings

Use fresh, thin shredded vegetables

3 lbs. of your favorite fish (without inner
   waste), boneless
1 cup sliced yellow squash (skin-on optional)
1 cup white tender shredded cabbage (raw)
1 large chopped onion
½ cup mixed sliced red and green bell
   peppers
½ cup chopped fresh parsley
1½ cups stiff cooked hominy grits
½ tsp. ground dill

Clean and scale fish well; be sure bones are removed, and
leave tail on. Season the inside and outside of fish. Spray
both inside and out with an olive-oil-flavored cooking spray.
Place all vegetables inside of fish. Wrap well with heavy foil,
leaving a small opening for steam to escape. Place in shal-
low pan. Add water at the bottom of pan. Cook over medium
high heat with cover for 35 minutes. Place warm grits all
over fish before serving.

The tail on the fish offers a good conversation topic at dinner time.

Old-fashioned Salmon with Herb Rice and Peppers
Yield 2 servings

1 cup canned pink salmon (undrained)

1 medium chopped onion

½ small green bell pepper, chopped

4 strips of lightly salted cooked hard bacon

1 cup cooked brown rice

1 tbsp. unsalted margarine

½ tsp. crushed dry rosemary

Check salmon for any little bones and excess skin.
Heat your skillet over a medium heat. Add margarine, peppers, onions, and rosemary.

Cook with lid on until tender. Fold salmon and rice into pan. Cook on low until heated through. Garnish with crumbled bacon.

Pink salmon, mackerel, and sardines in oil are great sources of omega three. Any of the three fish can be used for this tasty dish.

If your salt is completely restricted, disregard the bacon. Garnish with chopped fresh chives/sliced lemon.

Use rice often and make it brown. White rice is great, but brown is super-healthy.

Seafood Variety Patties
Yield 2 servings

8 oz. can of white tuna

½ cup flake white cooked fish

¼ cup imitation crabmeat, or original
   crabmeat

2 tbsp. light mayonnaise

1 tbsp. dry parsley

1medium diced onion

½ cup unsalted seasoned bread crumbs

Spray nonstick skillet with plain oil. Place over medium heat.

Combine in a medium-size bowl drained tuna, chopped crabmeat, fish, parsley, onions, and bread crumbs. Add mayonnaise and mix together. Form patties and cook.

Brown both sides.

Some shellfish is high in cholesterol and sodium. Continue to enjoy, but you have to practice portion control and variety.

Stuffed Devilled Shrimp
Yield 4 servings

4 hard-boiled eggs

12 cooked, cleaned, chopped medium shrimp

1 tsp. chili powder

1 chopped small red onion

1 tsp. fresh chopped parsley

1 tbsp. light ranch dressing

1 tbsp. hot sauce

1 tbsp. light mayonnaise

½ tsp. horseradish sauce

Cut eggs in half, lengthwise, remove yolks. Mix clean, chopped shrimp, onions, and dry seasonings. Add horseradish sauce, ranch dressing, mayonnaise and hot sauce; mix together well before adding to shrimp mixture. Stuff into each half of the hard-boiled egg whites.

If spice is not for you, omit it from recipe.

The title of the recipe is connected with the hot flavored ingredients.

Don't waste the egg yolks. Use yolks on the day regular eggs are allowed, on your favorite salad.
(Keep in a clean covered container - refrigerated.)

Creamed Fish/Corn
Yield 3 servings

6 oz. fish filet

½ tsp. dry dill

¼ tsp. white pepper

1 tsp. dry onion powder

Fresh parsley chopped

2 large slices marinated bell red peppers,
    chopped

11oz can cream corn

½ cup low-fat milk

1 cup chicken broth

1 tbsp. cornstarch

2 tbsp. unsalted margarine

Preheat skillet over medium heat. Add margarine.

Cut fish into 2-inch pieces. Season the fish with dill, onion powder, and pepper. Place fish in skillet and cook for 3 minutes a side. Remove fish from pan. Add peppers, corn, and broth. Mix in thickening made from milk and cornstarch. When desired thickness is obtained, add fish, remove from heat, top with parsley and cover.

This recipe may appear at first glance to be a long procedure, but don't be fooled.

Give that old tired fish recipe another kind of flavor. Use fresh parsley as one of your everyday herbs and onions for flavor.

CHAPTER TWO

SAVORY DRESSINGS AND STUFFINGS

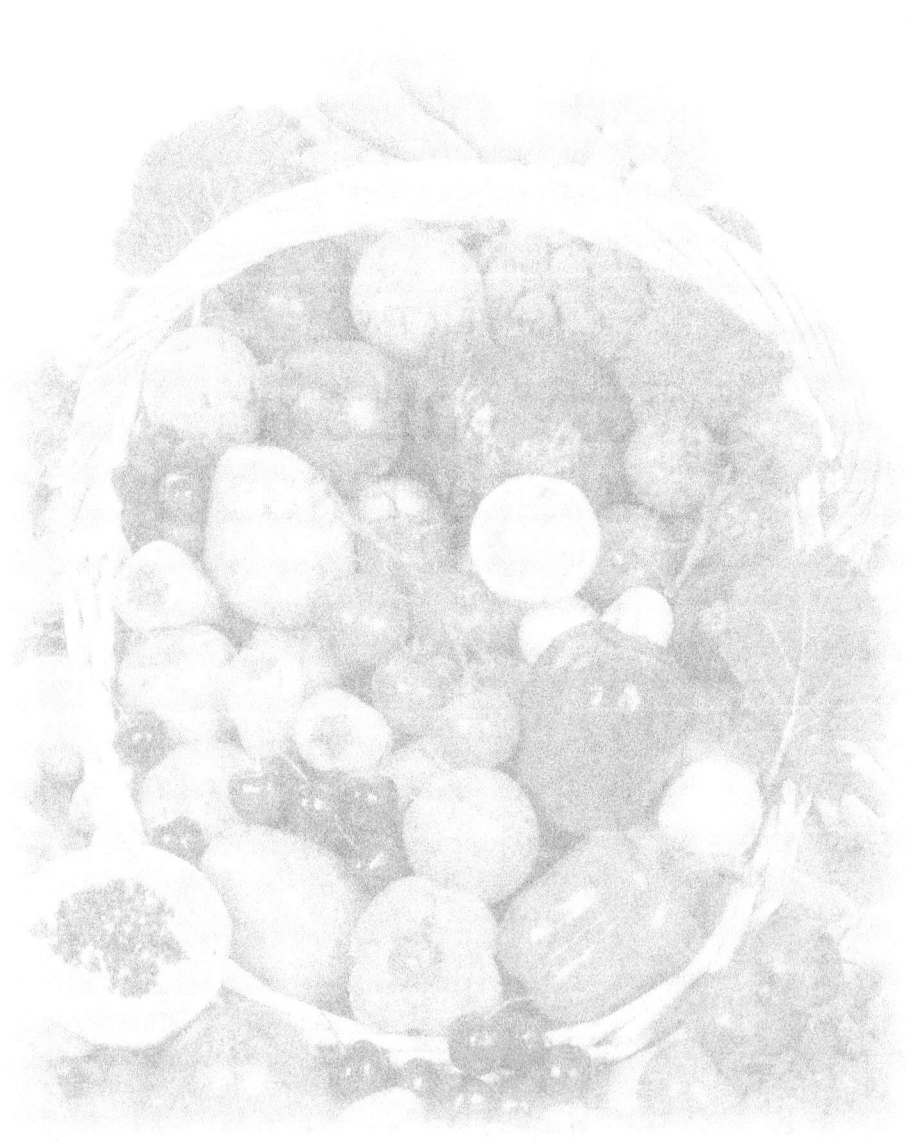

Vegetable Giblet Dressing
Yield 3 servings

4 slices wheat bread, 4 slices white bread
   toasted, spread with margarine and cubed

½ cup chopped sugar snap peas

½ cup diced broccoli (without flower) - just
   stems

½ cup green pepper

½ cup yellow pepper

1 large mild onion

3 celery stalks with tops on

1 small diced yellow squash (skin on)

1½ cup chopped giblets (gizzards, livers)

1 tsp. poultry seasoning

1 tsp. black pepper

2 tbsp. margarine

2 cups water

2 cups chicken broth

In saucepan over medium heat, add washed giblets, chopped celery and leaves, onion, bell peppers, water, and broth. Add snap peas, squash, and broccoli after giblets have cooked for 20 minutes. Let cook until gizzards are tender.

Remove from heat when done; strain, saving enough liquid to moisten dressing. In a bowl, place all vegetables and diced giblets, crouton-size toast that has been spread on both sides with margarine. Mix all ingredients together, re-check for correct seasoning desired. Place in a lightly buttered casserole dish. Place in preheated oven at 250 until top is crispy.

This dressing can be eaten as a meal, just by adding a few more oz. of protein. Since this recipe does consist of some cholesterol, be sure you use portion control, and all will be fine. Make sure if you add meat, the choice is lean. Reach back in the refrigerator for some of that leftover gravy.

Fruity Nutty Dressing
Yield 4 servings

8 slices nutty raisin toast

½ stick of unsalted margarine

½ cup mixed dry fruits (dry apricots, pears,
apples, figs)

½ cup diced carrots

¼ cup orange juice

½ cup chopped mixed unsalted nuts

Spread both sides of toast with margarine. Cut in crouton sizes. Add carrots, fruits and nuts; moisten with your favorite fruit juice. Place in buttered casserole dish. Let bake in preheated oven at 250 until top is dry.

This particular dressing can be used with any choice of meat or enjoyed just as is.

Hearty Grainy Vegetable Dressing
Yield 2 servings

1 cup cooked brown rice

2 cups chicken broth or stock

¼ cup unsalted sunflower seeds

½ cup cooked whole-kernel corn, drained

1 medium mild onion

½ cup diced celery

½ cup cooked, drained field peas

1 small yellow pepper

¼ cup margarine

Black pepper to taste

2 tsp. wheat germ

Cook celery, peppers, onion, and seasoning in broth. When done, drain; leaving a small amount of liquid for moisture. Add margarine, peas, corn, rice, and dry ingredients. Mix all ingredients together. Place uncovered in an oven-safe pan or dish in a preheated 200-degree oven. Let top get fairly dry, but not too hard to the touch.

Grandmom's Simple Stuffing
Yield 4 servings

8 slices day-old bread
1 medium onion
½ cup cooked diced celery
1 tsp. poultry seasoning
½ tsp. black pepper
3 tbsp. unsalted butter
1 cup of water

Butter both sides of bread. Cut bread in small cubes; add poultry seasoning, pepper, chopped clean celery, and onions, melted butter, and water for moisture.

When using butter or margarine, you must be careful. SATURATED FATS, TRANS FATS, AND CHOLESTEROL can be high. Practice reading your nutrition facts for your purchases. (Grand mom wouldn't cook without butter.)

This recipe is ready to stuff inside of your favorite poultry.

This recipe has been handed down for decades. Making it is quick, low cost and, with out a hassle. Don't be afraid to move your foods around in the same group. Just simple removal and replacement of foods can bring variety.

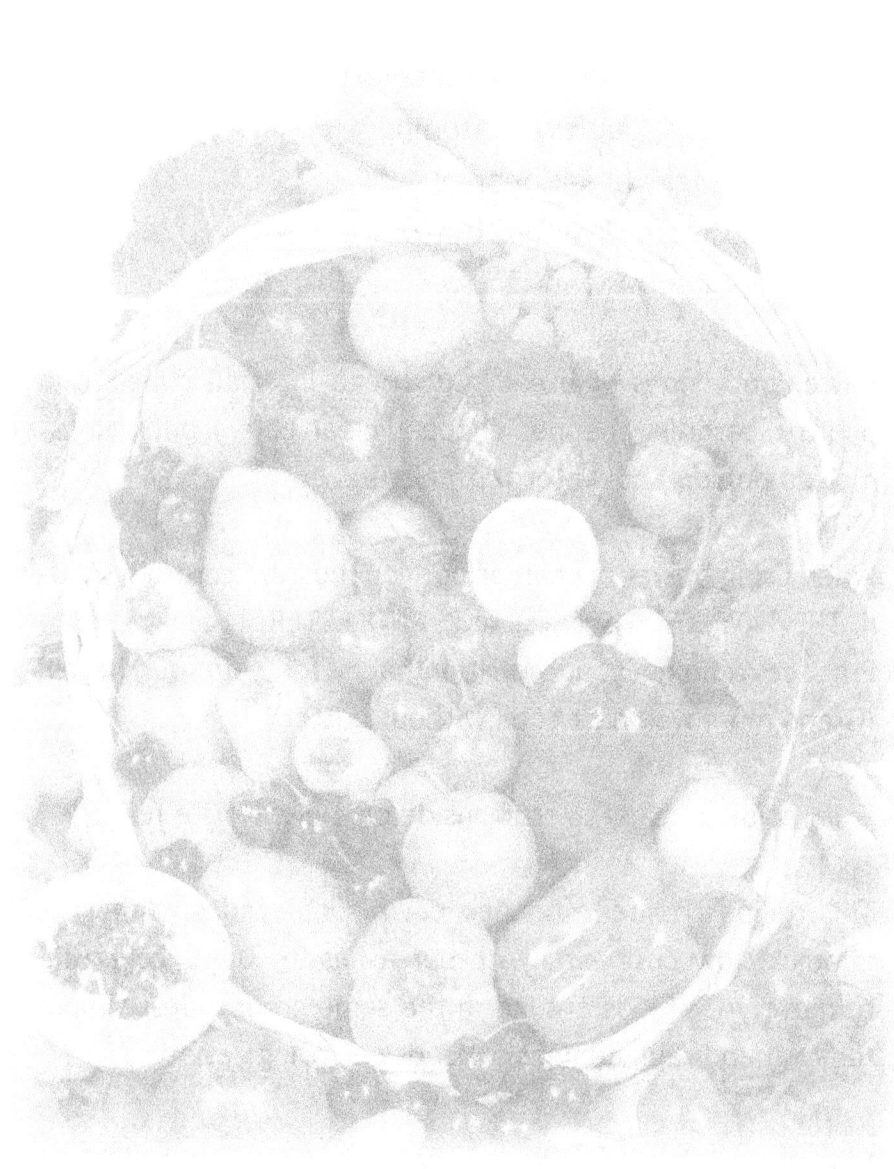

CHAPTER THREE

SALADS AND SOUPS

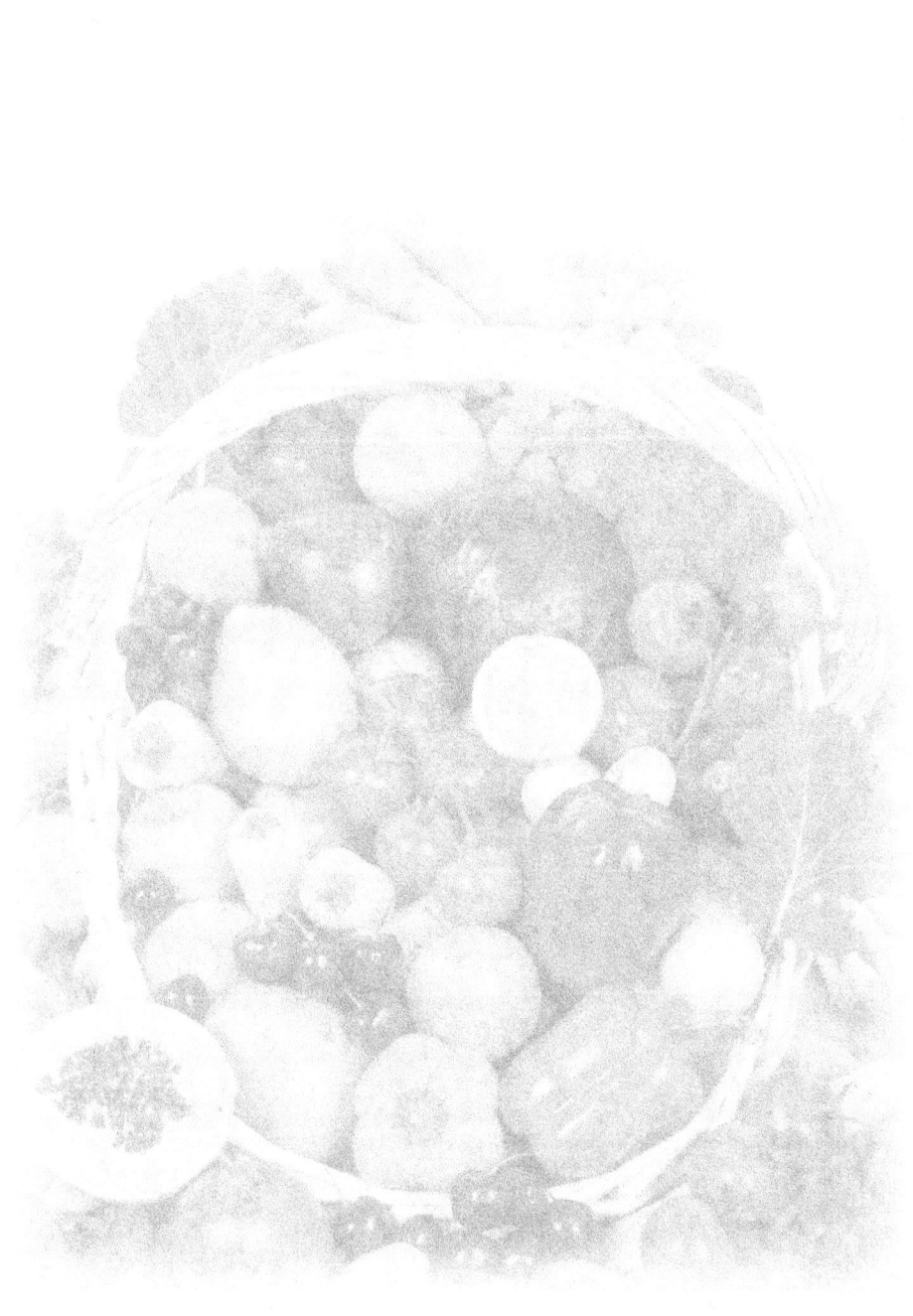

Stuffed Olives/Cucumbers
Yield 2 servings

12 green olives w/pimento

1 small sliced cucumber

4 whole medium or 6 small scallion bulbs

½ cup low-fat sour cream

1½ cups shredded red cabbage

Drain olives. Slice cucumbers thin with skin on. Clean, peel, and slice scallions being sure to remove the root tip. Blanche shredded cabbage in boiling water for a minute and place in ice cold water. Marinate olives, cucumbers, and scallions overnight in sour cream. Add to cabbage, toss and enjoy.

Keep your sour cream low in fat.

Assorted Nut/Apple Salad
Yield 2 servings

3 medium delicious apples
¼ cup shelled unsalted walnuts
¼ cup shelled unsalted pecans
¼ cup almonds
4 tbsp. light mayonnaise
1 tsp. lemon juice
8 whole lettuce leaves

Peel, core, and dice apples, and place in a large bowl. Add rough chopped nuts, lemon juice, and stir in mayonnaise. Serve over a bed of crisp lettuce.

These choices of nuts offer good nutrition: copper, zinc, vitamins, magnesium, calcium, and phosphorus.

At holiday time, put some of that nut assortment away for a salad day.

Sliced Tomato/Feta Cheese/Bean/Basil Salad

Yield 2 servings

3 medium tomatoes

½ cup dry feta cheese

1 can green beans

2 cups of favorite lettuce

¼ cup olive oil

½ cup green bean juice

¼ cup white vinegar

1 tsp of dried basil

Wash and slice tomatoes and assemble on a large salad plate. Add drained green beans. Mix together olive oil, vinegar, green bean juice, and chopped basil. Shake well; you have your salad dressing. Sprinkle cheese on top.

Practice using herbs as much as possible, instead of salty and fatty products.

Olive oil is a good fat, and our bodies welcome it in a small way. Foods and spices can be good and healthy; too much of a good thing can turn around and cause health problems.

Triple Red Salad

11oz can beets
1 large thin-sliced red onion
2 cups thin-shredded blanched red cabbage
1 bunch of parsley (washed well)
1 packet artificial sweetener
3 oz. apple cider vinegar
2 tbsp. canola oil
4 oz. beet juice

Place parsley as an under liner for your salad.

Drain and place beets over parsley on salad plate. Add a slice of thin round onions, and drained cabbage.

Mix beet juice, vinegar, sugar, oil. Shake well.

You are ready to enjoy a happy salad. Practice eating salads that offer green vegetables. Use dressings low in fat and salt.

Beets contain quite an amount of salt. Buy the low-salt canned style or go low on your serving size.

Potato Salad in a Shell
Yield 4 servings

4 small baking potatoes

1 small chopped onion

2 tbsp. sweet relish

2 hard-boiled chopped egg whites

1 tsp paprika

2 tbsp. light mayonnaise

1 tbsp. spicy mustard

Preheat oven to 400 degrees. Place potatoes in and cook until fork-done. Cut potato half, lengthwise and remove potato flesh keeping the skin intact. Put the skins aside. In a bowl, add all ingredients. Mix mayonnaise and mustard before placing into salad. Add remaining ingredients to potato flesh, stuff inside of potato skins, garnish with paprika, serve

Mustard contains salt; if kept at a small amount and not used too often, it shouldn't be a major problem.

Prune/Apricot/Peach Salad

Yield 2 servings

½ cup cooked prunes (pitted)

6 large unsweetened apricot halves, dry or
canned

1 cup unsweetened sliced peaches

2 tbsp. light cream cheese

2 tsp. sour cream

romaine lettuce hearts

Serve in small salad bowl cooled prunes, apricots, peaches;
top with cream cheese and sour cream. Garnish with chopped
lettuce. This salad is for two. Divide portions.

Apricots and prunes are full of potassium.

Vegetable/Cheese/Sage Soup
Yield 3 servings

1½ lbs. sage sausage

4 slices low-salt American cheese

2-10oz cans of condensed tomato soup

1 chopped medium onion

1 medium pepper (seeded and chopped)

1 cup skim milk

1½ tbsp. unsalted margarine

Brown the sage sausage in a nonstick skillet. (Drain off fat.) In a large soup pot over medium heat, add canned soup, milk, onions, and pepper. Add margarine, stir in cheese until incorporated with soup liquids. Add sausage last; stir, remove from heat, and cover.

Top with sage leaf before serving.

This is one of my latest soup recipes I found to contain a powerful group of flavors. I hope you find it the same. Tomatoes contain lycopene, an antioxidant that has been researched to be helpful to man's health problems that sometimes come in their later years. There are many other health benefits from this antioxidant. Use more tomato sauces in your meals. Vitamins A and C are high in fresh tomatoes.

Red Potato Soup
Yield 2 servings

4 medium red potatoes

3 scallions

2 cups chicken broth or stock

1 tbsp. chopped parsley

Wash and dice potatoes, leaving skin on. In a saucepan over medium heat, let broth become hot. Add diced potatoes, scallions, peeled and chopped fine, seasoning, and parsley. Cook until potatoes are tender.

This is loaded with potassium and perfect with a chef salad.

It doesn't take all day to eat happy and healthy.

Silky SMOOTH Cream
of CORN
Yield 2 servings

11oz can cream corn

½ cup soy milk

½ cup chicken broth

Cornstarch

1 package artificial sweetener

2 tbsp. margarine

Add milk, corn, and broth to blender and blend at medium speed for a minute. Remove. Place in saucepan over medium heat. Stirring, add margarine and sweetener. Remove 3 tbsp. of the corn mixture to thicken with cornstarch. Place cornstarch mixture in pot, stirring slowly until desired thickness. Add some seasonings if needed; it's great just the way it is.

This is easy, tasty, and no fuss.
So many of us these days are not allowed corn, nuts, and seeds. Whole corn is one of my favorite foods, so I found another way to enjoy corn.

Okra Onion Garlic
Turnip Soup
Yield 2 to 3 servings

½ lb. fresh or 1 small box frozen okra

2 fresh skinless chopped garlic cloves

1 chopped large onion

1 large turnip or 1 small box of frozen turnip

2 cups water

2 cups chicken broth

½ tsp. onion powder

½ tsp. garlic powder

Low salt seasoning

Using (fresh) cleaned diced vegetables, add all with seasonings to soup pot, over high heat. Bring to a boil and drop heat down to medium. Let simmer on low until all vegetables are tender.

For frozen-style, liquid should be hot before adding thawed vegetables. As you can see, using frozen foods can be quicker.

Okra is used in the Southern states as regularly as the northerners use peas, string beans, and carrots. A very nutritious choice, okra is loaded with vitamin C, low in calories and salt, and high in flavor.

Butternut Potato Soup
Yield 2 servings

2 cups frozen butternut squash (not mashed)

3 medium diced peeled white potatoes

1 medium chopped onion

½ tsp. nutmeg

2 tbsp. margarine

3 tbsp. skimmed ricotta cheese

½ tsp. black pepper

3 cups chicken broth

Over high heat, let broth, onions, pepper, and potatoes come to a boil. When potatoes are semi-tender, add squash and margarine (squash should be thawed). Cook until completely hot. Cover and remove from heat. Add a topping of cheese and nutmeg.

This squash is busting out with vitamin A and potassium. Sugar and salt are low, and flavor is high. Jump aboard and put squash on your grocery list regularly.

Beef-flavored Pasta
Soup
Yield 2 to 3 servings

2 cups elbow macaroni

1 medium red bell pepper

2 sliced cloves garlic

1 sliced, peeled, cooked medium taro root

3 cups beef broth

1 cup vegetable broth

1 tsp. onion powder

Using your soup pot, over high heat let broths, garlic, and onion powder, chopped cleaned peppers, seasoning, and taro root come to a boil. When taro root is tender, add pasta. Stir often until pasta is done. Meat doesn't have to be in a soup for it to be hearty.

Makes you want a second bowl!

Taro root is a veggie that can fit in the group with potatoes. This is mild in flavor with not as much starch. A great vegetable!

Try farmers markets for Taro Root

Mushroom/Bacon Soup
Yield 4 servings

2 cups of your favorite mushrooms

1 cup water

2 cups low-salt chicken or beef broth

½ cup each of onions and green peppers

4 strips lean turkey bacon

cornstarch

1 tsp. black pepper

½ cup shredded skimmed Muenster cheese

Put broth and water in medium pot. Cook over medium heat. When simmering, add mushrooms, onions, peppers, and seasonings. Make a thickener with liquid from soup and cornstarch. Add to pot and continue to cook over low heat. Stir often.

Cook bacon until crispy. Drain bacon on paper towel. Crumble and allow one strip for each 4 servings of soup. Top with cheese.

With most restrictions to certain foods, it is the amount eaten, not the food.

Continue to remove and replace where it is necessary for you. Soups can take little time and still give a shout of happiness.

Okra/Beef Soup
Yield 2 to 4 servings

2 cups frozen okra

2 cups frozen carrots

2 tbsp. low-salt margarine

3 lbs. cubed lean beef

1 large diced onion

2 cups shredded white cabbage

All purpose seasoning

1 tbsp. garlic powder

2 cups cooked brown rice

1 quart vegetable stock or broth

1 quart low-salt beef broth

You can use all fresh veggies. In your soup pot over medium heat, add liquids, washed beef, seasonings, onions, and cabbage.

Let pot heat covered. When beef becomes tender, add drained okra, carrots, margarine, and rice. Let pot remain covered on low heat.

When you use frozen vegetables or fruits along with fresh foods, always let your frozen foods thaw out before incorporating with each other.

Frozen vegetables in your menu planning, is a quicker way to get out of the kitchen without taking away from a happy, healthy meal.

Here is a perfect meal in one pot. Some mouth-watering desserts are soon coming up. Grab one to go along with this comforting meal.

Potato/Cheese/Celery Soup
Yield 4 servings

½ cup cream of potato soup (diluted)

1 cup cream of celery soup (diluted)

1 cup diced onion

1 cup diced Velveeta cheese

4 small cleaned skin-on red potatoes

½ cup chopped, cleaned fresh celery stalks

All purpose low-salt seasonings

1 quart low-salt chicken stock

Place soup and liquids in pot over medium heat. Stir until blended. Add onion, celery, and seasonings. When vegetables are tender, add cleaned, small, cubed potatoes. Add cheese when potatoes are fork-done. Stir until cheese is blended in well. If you need more thickness, add a small amount of cornstarch thickening.

Use cheese often in your meal-planning. It offers such good nutrition and flavor. Cheese doesn't just grab the attention of children; we enjoy it also. Use a cheese that blends well and also will stay smooth. Condensed soups contain salt; don't use too often in meal-planning.

You will notice onions are a very important part of my recipes. The onion offers awesome flavor. Choose good low-salt stocks and broths.

Curry Beef Soup
Yield 3 servings

3 lb. lean beef cubes

2 cups cooked kidney beans

1 large chopped onion

1 tsp. black pepper

2 tbsp. unsalted all-purpose seasoning

3 cups beef broth

3 cups water

2 tbsp. curry powder

3 stalks diced celery

1 cup tomato sauce

In soup pot, combine washed meat, diced onions, all dry seasonings, celery, water, and broth. Let cook covered until beef is tender. Add beans and tomato sauce. Continue to simmer until ready to serve. Garnish each serving with chopped chives.

Assorted Vegetable Soup
Yield 3 servings

Use a ½ cup each of frozen:

Brussels sprouts

Spinach

Diced carrots

Kale

1 large onion

Jarred artichoke hearts (drained)

3 cups chicken stock

3 cups water

½ tsp. black pepper

2 tbsp all purpose unsalted seasoning

Place liquids in soup pot over medium heat. Add diced onion, and pepper. Bring to a boil for 5 minutes. Reduce heat to medium and add drained vegetables. Let cook covered until all vegetables are tender.

Artichokes have their share of sodium. Vitamin C and iron are showing their face. An omelet and a crispy buttered roll would be just so good with this soup.

Vegetables are another doorway to good health. Fresh vegetables are best, and can be used in any recipe. The cooking time is longer.

Pork Pasta Onion Soup
Yield 2 servings

3 oz lean cubed cooked pork

2 diced large onions

2 garlic cloves, chopped fine, or 2 tbsp. garlic
    powder (optional)

1 large red bell pepper, cleaned and chopped

2 cups cooked elbow macaroni (whole-grain)

2 cups vegetable stock

2 cups chicken stock

1 cup water

All purpose salt-free seasoning

I recommend this recipe for most leftover meats. In soup pot over medium heat, add liquids, seasonings, onions, garlic, and red pepper. Let cook until onions are transparent. Add cooked meat and pasta. Cover pot and reduce heat to low.

Pork is a misunderstood meat. It gives ten necessary nutrients in a 3 oz serving of lean loin. The nutrients are dynamite, but there is sodium, cholesterol, calories, and other fats.

In order to take advantage of the nutrients offered, and not gather too much of the negativity, eat occasionally. Cook pasta in advance. Keep a small amount in the fridge. When you need it, it is ready.

Cream of Asparagus/Corn Soup
Yield 3 servings

3 cup cream of asparagus soup

1 cup pearl pre-cooked onions

1½ cups canned cream corn

1 cup frozen asparagus

2 cups chicken stock

½ cup skim milk

½ tsp. black pepper

1 small diced bell yellow pepper

Add to soup pot over medium heat: soup, stock, milk, cleaned pepper, and seasoning. Stir all ingredients until smooth. Cook until yellow pepper is tender.

Include drained asparagus, and drained onions. Add corn to pot and stir. Add cornstarch thickening if needed.

The market for frozen foods has become enormous. The recipes have been made to take less time in preparation for meals.

Asparagus is rich in vitamin B and other good nutrients.

Seafood Blend Soup
Yield 3 servings

1 cup crabmeat or imitation-style

1 cup cocktail shrimp

½ dozen mussels

2 medium large diced filet fish (any kind)

½ cup chopped fresh salmon

2 cups diced white potatoes

4 chopped whole scallions

2 cups chicken broth

2 cups mussel stock

2 cups water

1 tsp. seafood seasoning

1 tsp. crushed red hot peppers

This soup doesn't take a lot of time if you prepare it in sections. Day one, boil your mussels in 2 cups water or more. Remove from shell when done; leave in the liquid. All else can be done on the cooking day.

Place pot over medium heat. Add to mussel liquid and mussels other liquids, potatoes, chopped scallions, seasonings, and crushed peppers. When potatoes become fork-done, add fish, salmon, shrimp, and crabmeat. Continue to cook covered until desired done-ness. A large mixed green salad would be a perfect accompaniment to this tasty soup.

The broth is the best part of this soup. Perfect with a crusty roll.

Always tasty the next day.

Black and White Bean Soup
Yield 2 to 3 servings

2 cups of water

3 large fresh pre-cooked skinless turkey necks

1 cup cooked black beans

2 cups cooked navy beans

2 tbsp. onion powder

1 tsp. black pepper

6 cups low-salt chicken broth

1 large diced onion

This soup only needs to be heated well.

If you are not used to cooking this part of the turkey, you are in for a tasty surprise. Wash and skin necks. Place in pot with 2 cups water along with broth. Plenty of liquid will be necessary depending on turkey neck size. Add seasonings and onion. Cook for 2hours or until the meat separates from the bones. Add beans and enjoy. We all have our favorite soups; this will be an addition I am sure of this.

You can be healthy and still be happy.

How about a sandwich?

Use the best ingredients. The bread is the most important ingredient. The list of different kinds of breads offered now goes on and on. Look for breads made with WHOLE GRAIN. This provides the fiber needed in our diets and helps us with digestion.

Choose light dressings.

Pork Pita

Whole-wheat pita bread
Mixed greens
Spoon of applesauce
Sliced radishes
Provolone cheese
Sliced cooked pork loin

Push some leafy salad greens inside.

Pita breads are great choices for sandwiches.

PBF

On white toast, use a low-sodium creamy peanut butter. I prefer creamy, but chunky is all right too. Slice some sweet figs on top; a more grown-up twist to PBJ.

What a quick, tasty sandwich for the person on the run.

Super Fresh Vegetarian Sandwich

Soy sliced cheese
Eggplant
Yellow squash
Red onions
Cucumber
Black pitted olives

This is good way to use those grilled veggies. You can get grilled veggies from your supermarket or you can cook them at home. Use nutty wheat bread; start packing in the goodness. Add shredded Romaine lettuce, and tomato.

If you don't want to share, wrap half up well for another time.

Cheese/Fruit Open-face

3 tbsp. light cream cheese
4 large strawberries
1 medium banana
Whole wheat English muffins

This sandwich is great any time of day. It's quick, tasty, and really good.

Each serving is a half of toasted English muffin.

Each order has one sliced berry and 3 medium slices of banana.

This is a healthy choice, fiber from the bread, two fruits offering antioxidants and potassium, calcium in the cream cheese.

Be happy; make this sandwich a part of your AM or PM meal or a great night snack.

Overall, we all like a good sandwich. We just have to be a little more careful with the products we select to make them with. Do not use processed meats if you have a salt and fat problem. Fresh meat is the best way to go. Once in a while, put a small piece of a lean meat on to cook. Use it for making sandwiches on those days when going out is not on the schedule. Keep the dressing used low in fat and salt. At our age, we have a tendency to eat out a lot.

Keep in mind that bread products and fruits are also very necessary and important carbohydrates. All-natural products are super to use, just don't let the cost cause a financial problem. Sandwiches are not considered a meal unless it contains all the essential nutrition.

CHAPTER FOUR

FRUITS and VEGETABLES
The Backbone
Of Good Eating

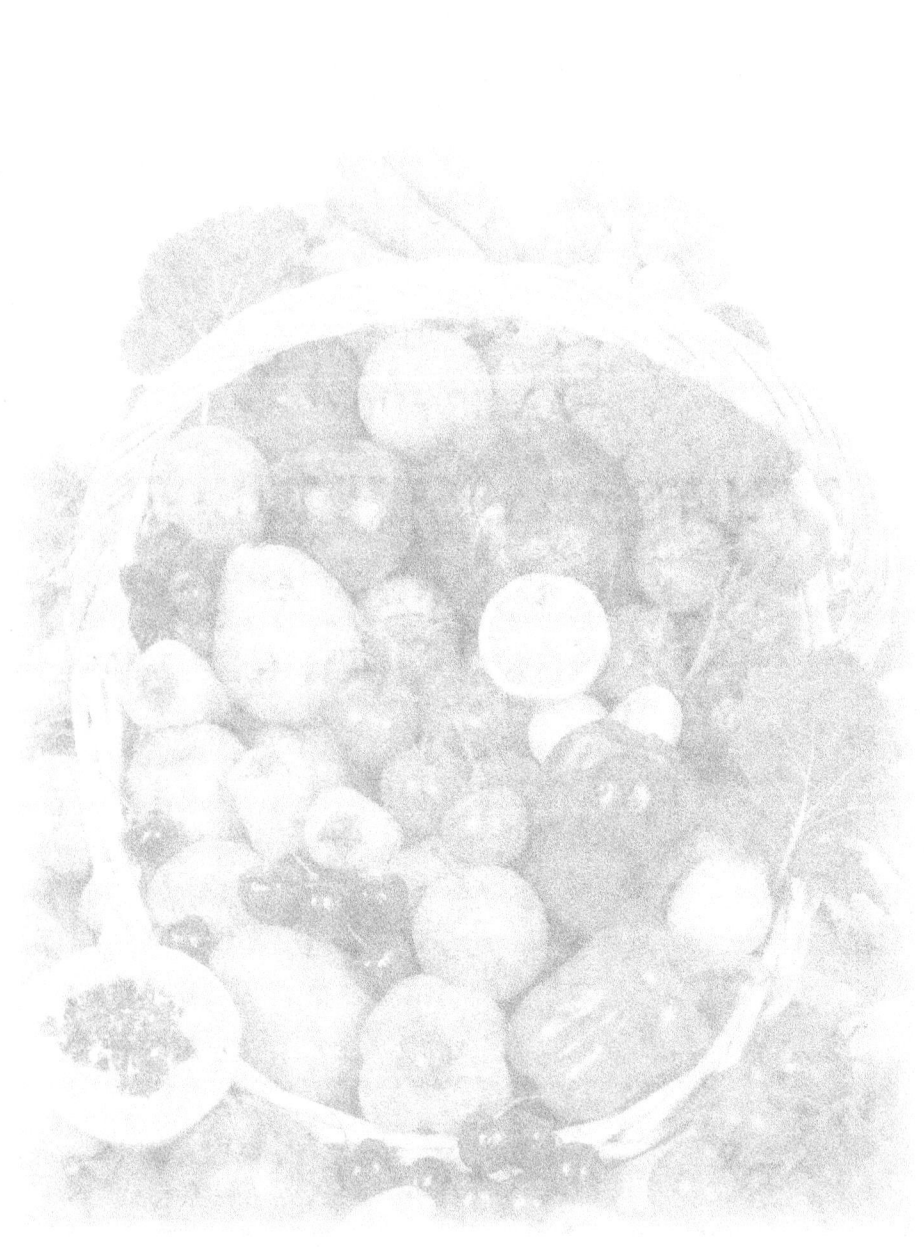

Fruit Stew
Yield 3 servings

2 medium hard apples

6 dry pitted prunes

6 dry apricot haves

2 figs

½ cup raisins

Cornstarch

1 medium hard pear

Low calorie sweetener

1 tsp. vanilla (imitation, or extract)

½ tsp fresh lemon

3 cups water

Wash all fresh fruits. Peel and core and remove pits from fruits. Cut into bite-size cubes. Add all fruits and seedless lemon, sugar, vanilla in given amount of water. Cook over medium heat until all fruit has softness. Remove fruits that become soft before others have cooked. When all fruits are done, remove from pot and set aside. Make a cornstarch thickening using juices from fruit. When desired thickness has been reached, cover and remove from heat. This is delicious with your favorite breakfast, or a midday snack.

Fresh and Canned Fruit Mixes
Yield 2 servings

½ cup diced canned unsweetened pears

2 medium diced apples

1 medium orange

½ cup canned unsweetened pineapple chunks

6 chopped fresh cherries

6 fresh dates

Peel and core apple; add pitted cherries, apricots; slice dates, peel orange sections and remove seeds. Combine all fruits, along with juice from pears, and pineapples.

Grab some in-between meals, for dessert at mealtime, for any reason, fruit is a winner.

A Sack of Goodness

2 medium sectioned fresh oranges
1 cup blueberries
3 tbsp. unsalted dry-roasted peanuts
2 peeled diced kiwi

Mix together in your favorite dessert dishes; sit back and enjoy.

This is something to keep you happy to nibble on while waiting for dinner.

Triple Tasty Greens
Yield 3 servings

½ lb. kale

½ lb. collard greens

½ lb. cabbage

3 cups low-salt chicken broth

1 large chopped onion

1 lb. sliced Italian sausage

½ cup chopped green bell pepper

½ tsp. black pepper

2 tbsp. unsalted seasoning

Wash all greens well and chop, but not fine. Include a piece of the core of the cabbage. Brown sliced sausage in soup pot. Add greens and seasonings. Cook over medium heat until greens become tender. Cover place on low heat until ready to eat.

The sausage is used for flavor; it may be removed. The salt and other flavors in the meat are what we need for this recipe. You can set the meat aside after it is cooked. It can be used in a dinner omelet in the near future (freeze it).

Three-Bean Pasta
Yield 2 to 3 servings

1 cup frozen green beans

1 cup frozen wax beans

½ cup canned French cut green beans drained

1½ cups cooked elbow macaroni

2 tbsp. unsalted margarine

Season to taste

1 tsp. chopped garlic (optional)

1 cup low-salt tomato sauce

2 medium chopped tomatoes

2 cups low-sodium chicken broth

Vegetables in this recipe are frozen already to combine. Place soup pot over medium heat. Add liquid, vegetables, beans, seasonings, margarine. Pasta and tomatoes go in last; stir well. Cover and let all ingredients heat.

Garnish this dish with a mixture of buttered flavored wheat croutons.

Keep in mind the dishes offered are to accompany needed protein. This dish is not completely nutritional enough in proteins to be a meal.

Cauliflower Supreme
Yield 2 servings

3 cups frozen cauliflower

1 cup frozen carrots

1 tbsp. low-fat sour cream

1 tbsp. unsalted margarine

1 cup shredded Lorraine Swiss cheese

1 cup diced cooked sweet potatoes

2 cups low-salt broth

In a saucepan over medium heat, let broth heat until hot. Add veggies, margarine, potatoes; season to taste. Stir in sour cream and cheese. Cover and keep on a low heat until cheese melts.

Lorraine Swiss is a mild-tasting low-fat cheese that can accompany most dishes and sandwiches. Sweet potatoes have been around for centuries. This is a naturally sweet and healthy starch. Potassium is related to this spud also.

Eggplant Delight
Yield 2 servings

1 large eggplant

½ cup skim pepper jack cheese

1 medium sliced onion

1 tbsp. canola oil

1 medium sliced red bell pepper

1 cup cream of chicken soup (diluted)

1 tsp. black pepper

All-purpose low-salt seasoning

½ cup herb-flavored croutons

1 cup water

Preheat skillet over medium heat. Add oil, onions, and peppers. When tender, drain pan of extra juices. Add soup and water to pan. Stir, place peeled eggplant sliced 2 inches thick.

Cook until tender. Place cheese all over top of eggplant delight.

Top with herb-flavored croutons.

Vegetables and fruits play a large part in keeping the scale of good nutrition leveled. Fit it into your daily meal planning. Eat a variety every day. In order to get the advantage of the different nutrients they give, you have to keep the circle constantly turning.

Good choices of cheeses can give you protein and calcium in a big way without the unneeded fats, salt, and cholesterol. A food can be healthy, but overeating can make it become unhealthy.

Creamed Beets And Peppers

1 can of sliced beets

6 whole pearl onions

1 tbsp. sour cream

2 tbsp. margarine

1 small yellow and 1 red bell pepper

1 cup low-fat milk

2 cups water

1 tbsp. cornstarch

Over medium heat in a non-stick saucepan add onions and chopped peppers. When tender, add sliced canned beets, margarine, and seasoning. Remove a couple large spoons of beet juices; mix with cornstarch until mixture is smooth. Replace in pot, stirring until all is blended and thickened to your approval. Remove from heat and cover.

As delicious as they are, keep in mind that beets can be high in sodium.

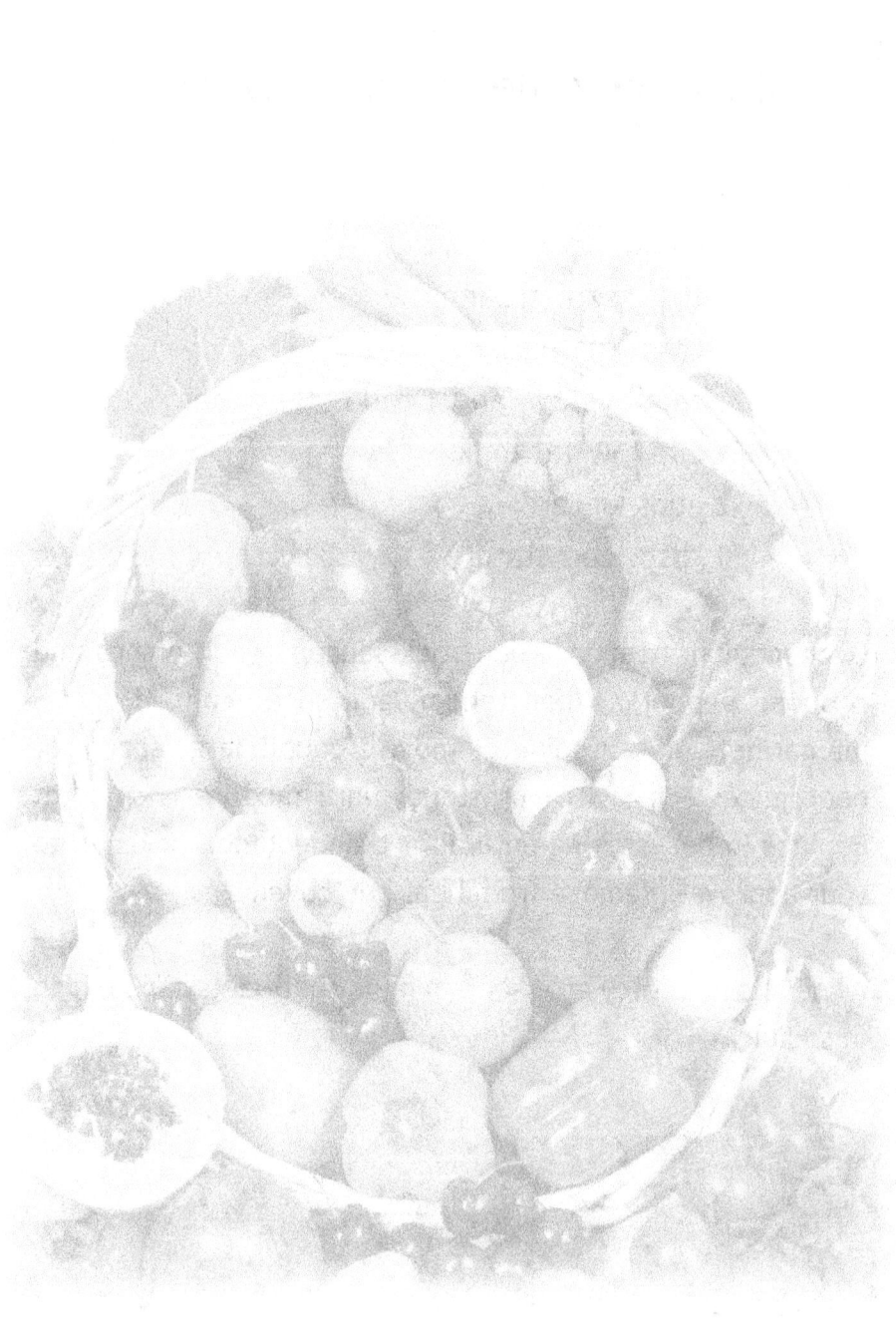

CHAPTER FIVE

ENJOY YOUR DESSERTS
Without The Sugar And Fat

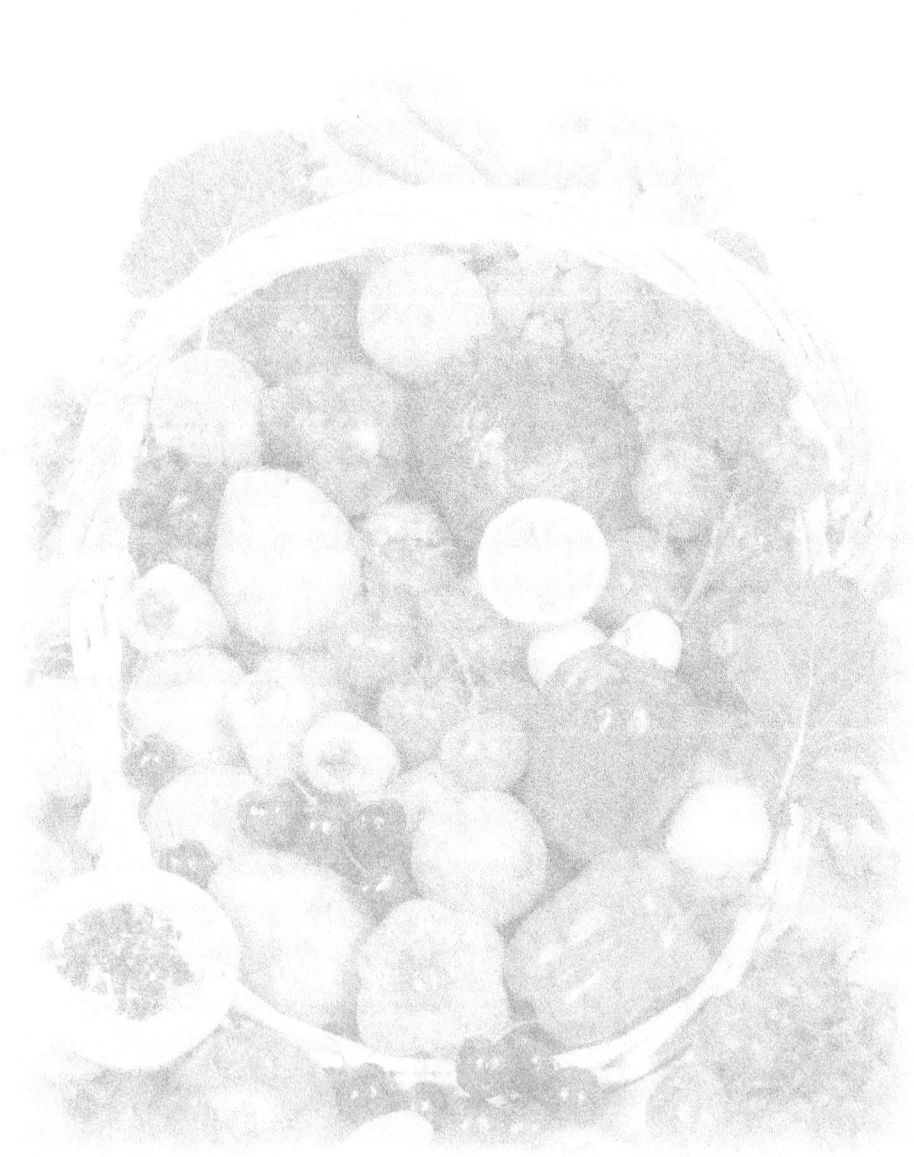

When preparing desserts, you have to use the products that your diet calls for. Desserts mostly consist of fats, sugars, and starch. These can be trouble, so portion control is a must in all restricted meal planning. The following recipes can be rearranged to fit both regimen styles of meal planning: house style and restricted style. All foods used are low in fats, sugar, and cholesterol and salt. If you are allowed sugar, use it. If your cholesterol is at a good level, practice keeping it there. Removal and replacement is all it takes for all to enjoy the following desserts

These delicious, mouth-watering desserts were made with you and me in mind.

In order for any healthy menu planner to work being honest to your self is the key.

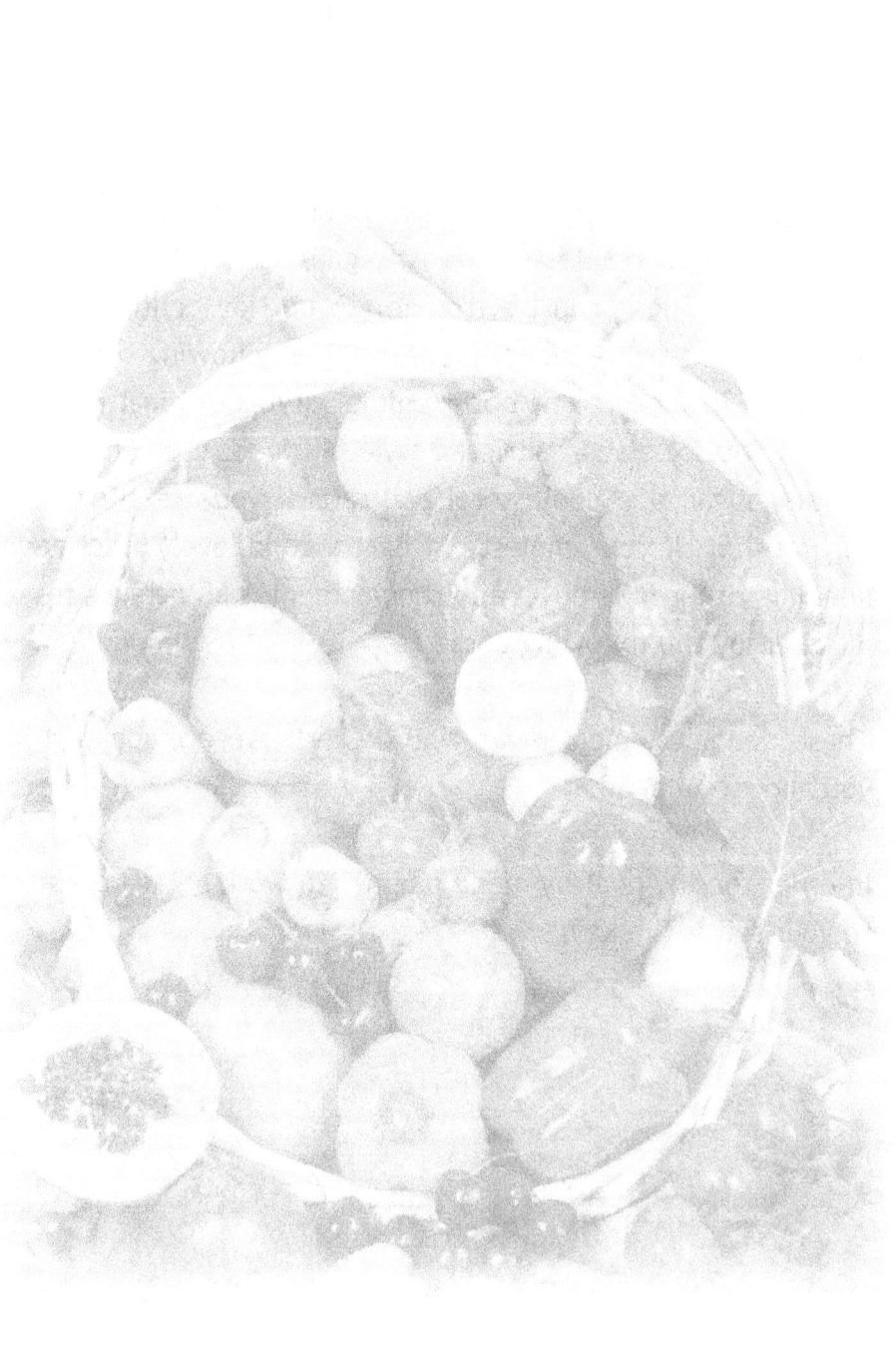

Cherry/Jubilee
Yield 2 servings

Sugar-free fat free ice cream (2 oz. per
   serving)
1 regular-size junior baby cherries (baby
   food)
4 small low-sugar, low-fat cookies
2 dark chocolate almond kiss candies

Place 2 ounces of ice cream, your choice of flavor, in a serving dish. Garnish with crumbled cookie and top with 1 tbsp.
of baby cherries. Top with a kiss.

This dessert is low in sugar and fats. If you have a high glucose count, you had better pass this arrangement up. If
your blood count is controlled and you stick to given recipe
amounts without eating a large amount of fats and starches
with your meals, give yourself a treat. This type of dessert is
not recommended every day or every week. Portion control
has to be visible in order to be successful on any diet regimen.

Chunky/Hunky Nutty Fruit
Yield 2 to 3 servings

1 cup chunky honeydew melon

1 cup chunky cantaloupe

1 cup watermelon

½ cup chopped unsalted mixed nuts

2 pkgs. artificial sweetener

1 tsp. banana flavoring

Mix fruit in large bowl. Mix flavoring, sugar, and nuts; blend in with fruit. Let chill and serve.

A variety of fruits is needed daily. Make sure you don't lean toward the ones high in natural sugar too often

Tapioca Goodness
Yield 2 servings

2 cups tapioca
½ tsp. cinnamon
1 tsp. vanilla flavor
1 cup mandarin oranges
¼ cup low-fat milk
4 unsalted pretzels

Stir in vanilla flavoring, cinnamon, and milk to tapioca. Fold in drained oranges.

Place in dessert dishes and chill. Garnish with pretzels, when ready to serve.

Always choose snacks with low sugar and salt and fat in mind.

Rum-Flavored Rice Pudding
Yield 2 to 3 servings

2 cups cooked rice

½ tsp. rum flavor

½ tsp. nutmeg

1 cup low-fat sugar-free vanilla pudding

½ cup low-fat and low-sugar whipped cream

½ cup low-fat milk

In a large bowl, mix rice, vanilla pudding, nutmeg, flavoring, and milk; stir well. Fold in whipped cream. Chill.

Peanut Butter/Applesauce Spread with Raisins

Low-fat peanut butter (all-natural)
½ cup unsweetened cinnamon applesauce
2 halves of raisin English muffins

Split and toast muffins; add allowed amount of peanut butter and applesauce.

Oh boy! tasty, quick, and healthy. So why shouldn't you be happy?

Yogurt With A Fling
Yield 2 servings

1 cup vanilla-flavored yogurt

2 small ginger muffins

1 medium banana

½ cup unsweetened granola

2 chopped figs

2 tbsp. sugar-free maple syrup

2 tbsp. low-fat milk

Using a blender, add milk, yogurt, sliced bananas, granola, figs, and maple syrup.

Blend until semi-smooth. Pour over your muffin, or just dip.

Good source of roughage. This is a very good way to start your day.

Blanket of Snow
Yield 2 servings

2 slices cinnamon-raisin bread
2 large beaten egg whites
1 pkg. artificial sweetener
2 tbsp. low-fat whipped cream

Preheat a nonstick skillet on medium heat. Spray skillet with butter flavored cooking spray. Mix sweetener to egg whites. Dip bread in egg batter, and place in skillet. Let cook until both sides are brown. When cool, cover with whipped cream.

Don't get too excited; it's just your usual French toast with my flair.

Nutty Cream

4 tbsp. low-fat cream cheese

¼ tsp. almond flavor

6 low-sugar shortbread cookies

½ cup each small fresh diced apples and
    pears

¼ cup pre-soaked raisins in warm water

¼ cup apricot nectar

Add flavoring to cream cheese; combine all fruits and juice.

A perfect spread for your cookies or crackers.

The "nutty" is in the flavoring.

Kiss of Chocolate
Yield 3 to 4 servings

¼ cup dark chocolate chips

3-4 oz. dessert dishes

1 box sugar-free cherry Jell-O (regular size)

Follow directions on Jell-O package.

Place a few chocolate chips in the bottom of dessert dish. After Jell-O has cooled, add to dishes and chill until jelled.

Dark chocolate is healthy; we make it unhealthy by overeating.

Strawberry Peanut Butter Grahams
Yield 3 servings

6 graham cracker squares

3 tbsp. peanut butter

3 tbsp. sugar-free strawberry preserves

Add 1 tbsp. peanut butter on three of the squares, and preserves on the other three.

Put them together, and what a delicious treat, and you have some protein going on.

Perfect for a midday snack.

Pancake Wrap

3 large, thin pancakes
3 tbsp. preserves
3 tbsp. low-fat sour cream

The next time you make pancakes, make the batter thin. After pancakes are done, cool, add one tbsp. preserves and one of sour cream, and roll up. Use your favorite preserves; the choices are many. Grab one when you have that early-morning appointment. Wrap and go.

Banana/Peach Twirl
Yield 4 servings

1 jar junior-style baby bananas

1 medium banana, sliced

4 unsweetened peach halves

1 cup low-fat tapioca pudding

½ cup low-fat whipped cream

In 4-oz. dessert dishes, add 1 peach half, 2 tsp. baby bananas, whipped cream, and a few slices of banana.

I recommend using baby foods whenever fruit is allowed. It also provides the needed nutrition. Baby foods are perfect for cream soups, sauces, gravies, and desserts. What is happier and healthier than a well-fed baby?

Warm Apple Rice Pudding.
Yield 3 servings

Core and skin 3 medium golden delicious apples. Shred and add to your favorite rice pudding. Warm for 2 minutes, covered, in the microwave. When you buy your rice pudding, do not be afraid to add your choices to the pudding.

When you choose a starch for dessert, make sure your main meal wasn't planned with extra starches.

Strawberry Peach Fig Pudding
Yield 4 servings

½ cup each sliced figs, strawberries, fresh or
    sliced peaches
20 vanilla wafers
1 cup low-fat sugar-free whipped cream
2 cups low-fat sugar-free vanilla pudding

In a deep bowl, mix all fruits. Add pudding to each dessert dish; top with fruits, then cookies 2 each layer. End with whipped cream. Repeat until three layers have been made. Garnish complete top with a whole strawberry and cookie. Chill.

It is important to serve your desserts with the correct serving size. This helps us not to overload, and stay within the proper portion. You never make too much; put away for the next time. Some foods are not used in recipes as much as others figs and dates are a few.

This recipe will give four people a dessert that they will tell their doctors about!

This dessert is so satisfying and delicious you will not believe your glucose can be safe. If you have any doubt with any recipe, check with your medical team first.

Please give the proper information.

Brown Bombers
Yield 4 servings

4   2-inch brownies
4   2-oz. sugar-free fat-free chocolate yogurt
½ cup low-sugar low-fat chocolate pudding
½ cup sugar-free fat-free chocolate whipped
    cream

Place 1 brownie on top of 2 ounces of yogurt. Top with a small spoonful of pudding. Top with small spoonful of low-sugar low-fat chocolate whipped cream.

The market is very large in offering the sugar- and fat-watchers condiments and many other essential needs. The health stores have expanded enormously. If you look in the correct areas, you can find 90 percent of your meal-planning needs.

Mixed-berry Shortcake
Yield 3 servings

1 cup blueberries, strawberries, blackberries
   (frozen fresh)
3 slices angel food cake
½ cup low-fat whipped cream
2 pkgs. artificial sweetener

Place frozen berries with sweetener added overnight in re-frigerator.

Add 1 heaping tbsp. of fruits and juices over cake. Top with whipped cream.

A good dessert to make when the grandchildren come over!

Chocolate Upset
Yield 2 servings

2 cups sugar-free low-fat dark chocolate
   pudding
6 sugar-free low-fat chocolate cookies
3 tbsp. low-salt cashew butter
3 tsp. marshmallow whip

Spread cashew butter on each cookie. Chop with a knife to crumble slightly.

Place in dessert dishes, add pudding, let chill. Garnish with marshmallow whip.

Jarred marshmallow can be purchased low in sugar.

Coffee Mellow
Yield 3 servings

3 2-oz. servings sugar-free low-fat vanilla
ice cream

6 oz. decaf coffee

3 tsp. whipped cream, low-fat and sugar-free

2 pkgs. artificial sweetener

In 4-oz. dessert dishes, add ice cream, coffee sweetened with sweetener, and whipped cream.

Save the unused coffee; it will stay well-chilled.

Sweet Potato Coconut Whip

3 medium sweet potatoes

½ tsp. vanilla flavor

½ tsp. lemon flavor

Low calorie sweetener

3 tsps unsalted margarine

½ cup low-fat milk

2 tbsp. dry coconut

Boil potatoes with skin on over high heat. Peel when cooled. In a mixing bowl, place sliced potatoes. Add melted margarine, milk, and flavoring. Using mixer, beat until all ingredients are blended. Add sweetener to taste. Place in dessert dishes, and add coconut. This can be eaten chilled or at room temperature.

Dry Coconut can be purchased unsweetened.

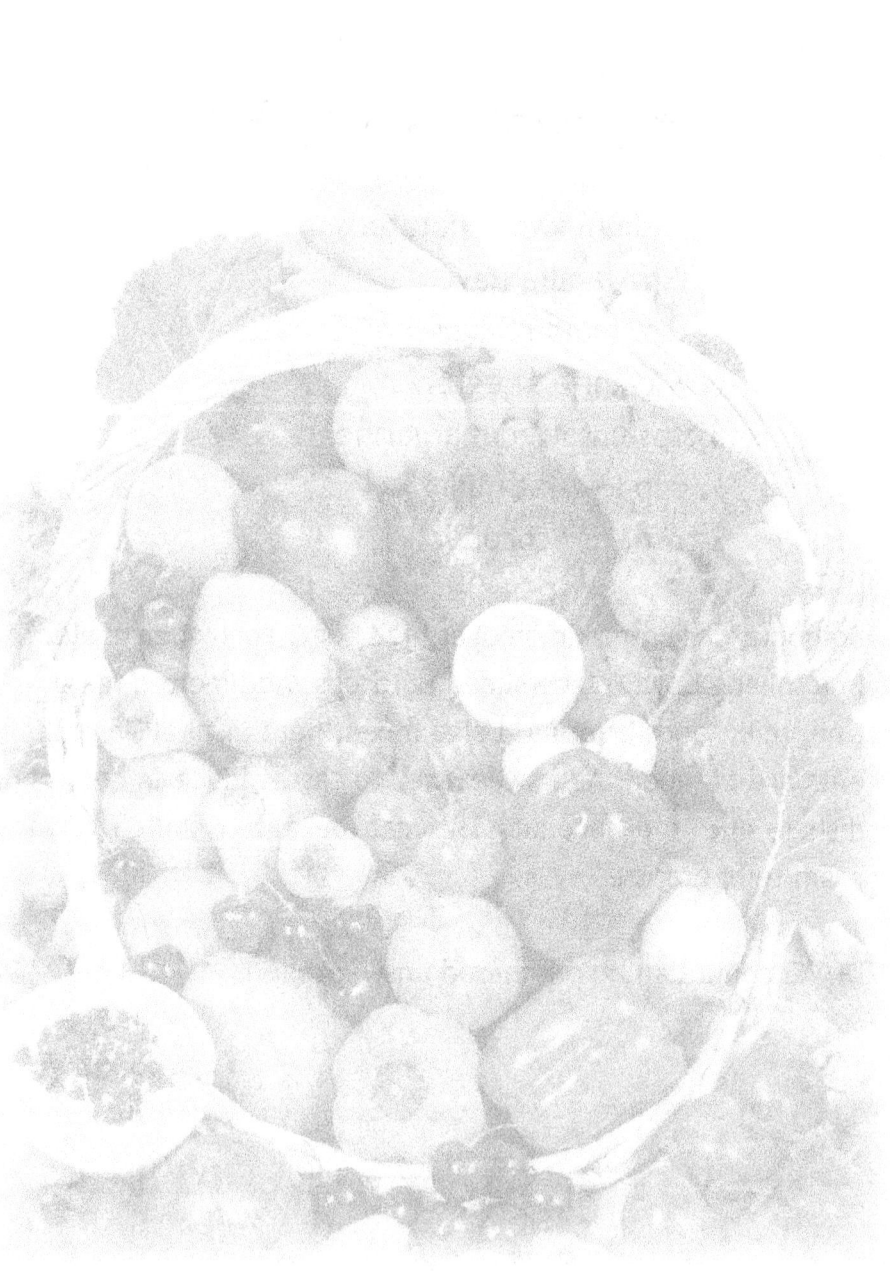

CHAPTER SIX

PUTTING IT ALL TOGETHER

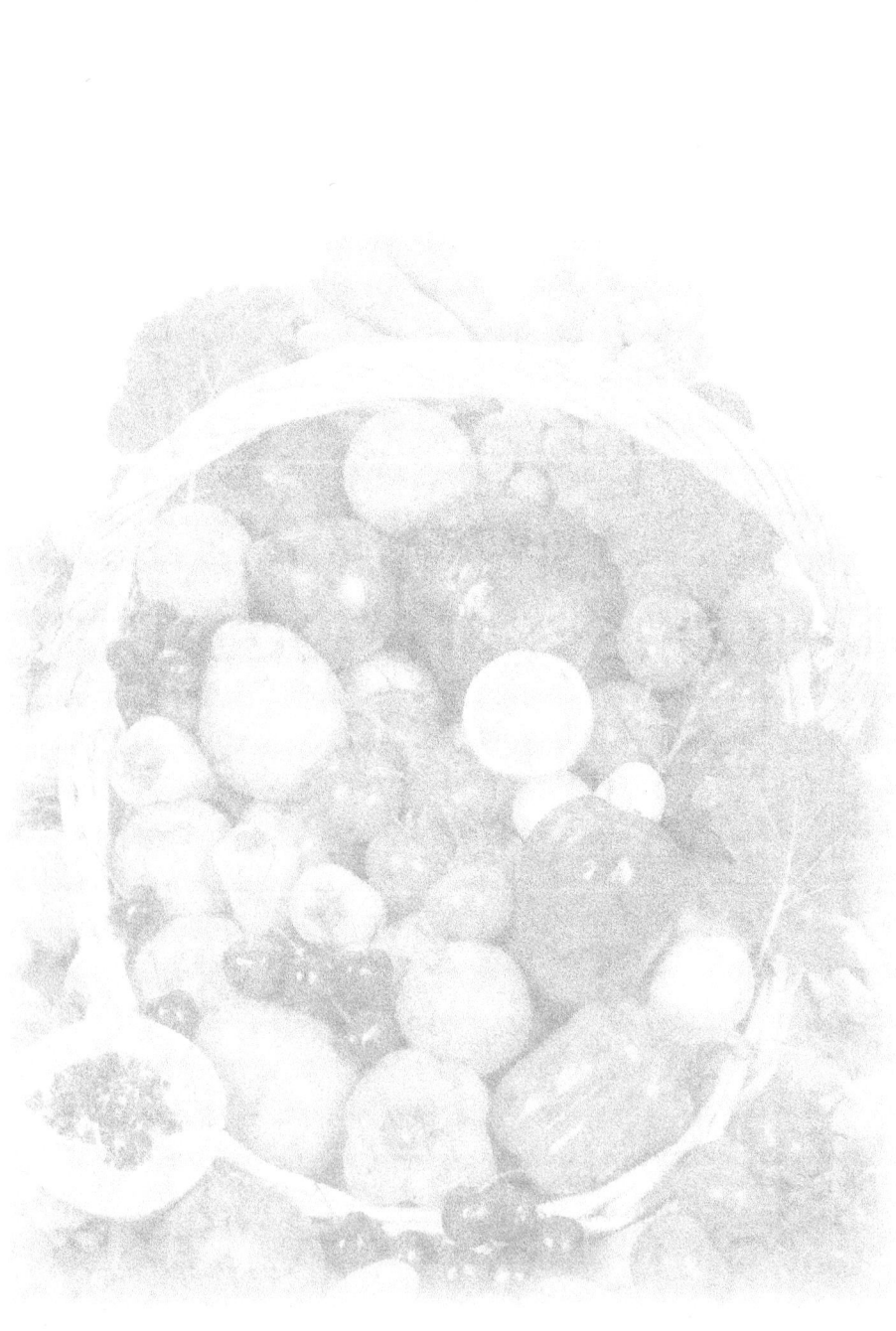

Meal Planning

To have healthy, happy meals, make sure your choice of foods have nutritional value along with taste. All your meals should be welcomed with great anticipation. Don't get to the point where looking forward to eating is like dreading a pain on the way. I am bringing you recipes that will give you flavor, and are a pleasure to sit down to. Wise meal-planning results in a healthy, happy meal. Food is eaten for the maintenance of the body; it should also offer contentment and relaxation. Someone made a remark in my presence, "What's the big deal?" The deal is, because we have restrictions, why should our meals be blah? We are seniors, which is an age, not a condition. Try the trade system in meal planning: 1 tsp. oil = 1 slice bacon; 1 egg = 1 oz. lean meat. The nutritional value has to be the same for a proper trade. Fit milk or milk products into your daily meals. If you get bored from plain milk, try the different flavors of milk coming up later that are simply full of flavor. The following meals are just to show how it can be done.

Although we have much in common in meal planning, being aware of your own boundaries is what is important. Don't follow a friend's meal portions. Their's may be 1800 calories a day, and yours 1500 calories a day. You can have the same food issues, but on different levels of needs.

Breakfast with Mid-morning Snacks

No egg yolk products are used.

½ cup per serving for cereals.

No more than one slices of any bread per meal.

#1

Fish/hominy grits (2 ounces fish/2tbsp hominy
   grits on top)

Wheat toast/margarine

Stewed fruit

Hot beverage

Milk

Snack — Jell-O

#2

Creamed chipped chicken/hard toast

Warm stewed fruit

Hot beverage

Snack — graham crackers/milk

#3

Cottage cheese

Sliced fried tomatoes

½ English muffin/toasted

Nutty fruit

Milk

Snack — unsalted vegetable chips/fruit juice

#4

Cream wheat /non-dairy cream
Egg Beaters
Rye toast/light cream cheese
Assorted fruit
Hot beverage
Snack — milk/tapioca pudding

#5

Fluff/Buff omelet
Cinnamon toast/applesauce
Juice
Snack — cold cereal/milk

#6

Beef potato pancakes
Ketchup (low salt, low sugar)
Fruit
Milk
Snack — milkshake

#7

Small lean pork roll
Raisin toast/margarine
Juice
Hot beverage
Snack — hot chocolate/fruit

#8

Steamed rice/eggs/cheese

Tomato juice

Hot beverage

Snack — slice melon

#9

Open-face soy cheese melts

Granola/fruit

Hot beverage

Snack — pudding/cookies

Hey! We are not ready to stop going yet. We are active and on the go with our center visits and other hobbies. Try one of my original healthy, happy drinks. Pull out the blender!

Strawberry-Banana Float

8 oz. skim milk
½ cup sliced strawberries
½ sliced small banana
1 tbsp. whipped cream
Low calorie sweetener

Blend and chill.

This is a good way to also use your fruits in a happy way.

An Apple A Day ...

½ cup cored diced apples (skin off optional)

4 oz. apple juice

4 oz. low-fat milk

¼ cup shredded fresh carrots

Blend on high, chill, and enjoy.

Nutty Eggnog

8 oz. low-fat milk

1 oz. Egg Beaters

Ground mixed unsalted nuts

¼ tsp. vanilla flavor

½ tsp. nutmeg

1 tbsp. low-fat, unsweetened whipped cream

1 packages low calorie sweetener

Blend and chill.

Apricot-prune Whip

½ cup apricots with juice
6 oz. low-fat milk
4 pitted, chopped prunes
Low calorie sweetener

Blend and chill.
Blend drinks semi-smooth.

Merry Berry Drink

¼ cup of each blackberries, strawberries,
    blueberries
8 oz. skim milk
2 tsp. light whipped topping
Low calorie sweetener

Blend and chill.

Ice is not needed in any of the above drinks. Unsweetened,
low-fat, low-cholesterol whipped creams only are used. Artificial sweeteners only.

The above are my special choices; feel free to make yours.
This is how new recipes arise.

A Chocolate Lift

4 oz. skim chocolate milk
4 oz. skim milk
4 unsweetened chocolate chips
½ tsp. vanilla flavor
 sweetener to taste
½ cup sliced fresh strawberries

Blend and chill.

Keep your unused fruits in a well-sealed container in a cool place. If you are allowed more fruit, go ahead and pile in that vitamin C.

Pineapple Whisper

½ cup drained chunky pineapple
½ cup drained mandarin oranges
4 oz. sugar-free ginger ale
4 oz. cranberry juice
Low calorie sweetener

Blend and chill in freezer.

This is another way to use fruits when you have had your milk quota.

Grapes And More Grapes

12 seedless red grapes
12 seedless black grapes
12 seedless white grapes
6 oz. grape juice
4 oz. apple juice

Blend well and chill's you enjoy the skin of the grape; there's no need to strain the juice. We all can use fiber now and then. This drink is not only packed with flavor but also solid nutrition.

A Sunshine Drink

½ cup orange juice

½ cup diced fresh or canned peaches

4 chopped dry apricots

4 oz. unsweetened pineapple juice

¼ cup diced mango

Low calorie sweetener

Blend and chill.

Snow Ride For Two

16 oz. coconut milk

½ cup unsweetened dry coconut

3 tbsp. whipped cream

2 4-oz. dips sugar-free vanilla frozen yogurt

1 tsp. vanilla flavor

Blend well and chill.

If you have a problem in digesting raw coconut, omit.

Being honest with you; we all know our allowances. If you are allowed only ½ cup milk, 1 fruit each meal, the above drinks can accommodate most allowances for a meal. Any you have left over, keep chilled for no more than a couple days. You don't want to lose too much of the nutrients.

Keep a good count of your fruit amounts and portions. There are many ways to use your fruits besides just directly just eating them as is. Mix and match these delicious and quick drinks with your meals and snacks. You will be eating fruit allowances and more. Be careful.

Lunch Meals and Midday Snacks

#1

Beef broth
Tuna salad stuffed in wheat pita bread
Fruit
Beverage
Snack — vanilla wafers/milk

#2

Chicken broth
Open-face toasted muffin/grilled hamburger
Cole slaw
Snack — Apricot shortcake/milkshake

#3

Okra Celery soup
Stuffed deviled shrimp/romaine lettuce
Unsalted assorted crackers
Lime aide
Snack — fruited Jell-O/milk flavored drink

#4

Fruit/cottage plate/nut bread
Hot side dish buttered carrots
Cherry lemon hot tea
Snack-1/2 fresh turkey sandwich/
    mayonnaise/fruit juice

#5

Black/White Soup

Mixed green tossed salad/dressing

Fresh fruit in season

Milk

Snack — low sugar frozen yogurt

#6

Tomato soup

Pork/rice salad

Pudding

Hot lime/kiwi tea

Snack — apple/cheddar cheese

Choose your lunch according to what your dinner will be. Stay in your boundary of calories and other allowances the best you can. Be constant in your battle. Remember you are joined with many in your struggle to eat for health.

Dinner

You are about to have what many people consider the most relaxed meal of the day. Each day, all three snacks can be taken from previous meals. This comes under the heading of foods left over. I find foods taste even better after sitting a day or two in the correct environment. Making dinner extra tasty and mouth-watering is exciting; the healthy will be there also because you choose the correct foods, prepared and cooked right for you.

Be sure to include snacks in your meals, if you have been told to.

#1

Beef jubilee

Creamed beets and peppers

Fruit juice

Hot beverage

Snack — strawberry peanut butter grahams/ milk

#2

Creamed fish and corn

Croutons flavored with margarine

Fig nut salad

Snack — unsalted air-popped corn/Sunshine drink

#3

Sauerkraut/steamed loin chop/apples

Mashed potato

Parsley carrots

Plum pudding

Milk

Snack —fresh fruit

#4

Butternut soup

Baked chicken/peaches

Seasoned kale

½ slice bread/margarine

Fruit juice

Snack — Hot pineapple-flavored tea/½ light
    cream cheese sandwich

#5

Mint and cranberry-flavored lamb chops

Spinach/goat cheese

Brown/rice

Fruited Jell-O

Snack — Cold cereal/milk

#6

Red potato soup

Sliced roast beef/mushrooms

Buttered broccoli/ricotta cheese

Stewed tomatoes

Hot beverage

Snack — caramel-flavored milk/peanut butter
crackers

#7

Low salt vegetable juice

Veal Italia

Mixed fruit juice

Hot beverage

Snack — sweet potato coconut whip/milk

#8

Old-fashioned salmon/herbal rice

Garlic/olive-flavored French green beans

Lemon hot tea

Snack — pineapple cheese cookies/milk

#9

Turkey broth

Assorted salad greens, marinated with
vegetable oil dressing. Topped with
assorted cheeses/diced beets/marinated
red bell peppers.

Unsalted assorted wheat and oat crackers

Fruited yogurt

Snack — Merry Berry milk/graham crackers

Your choices for dinner don't always have to be what society has stamped "just for dinner." Any foods that are enjoyable to you should be what your menu should be. What is wrong with a Fluff and Buff omelet for dinner? Like I said earlier, add more protein or vegetables, if this is what is needed to make the choice good for you. I hope that everyone who reads my recipes can obtain nothing but good responses. All recipes were made with seniors first in mind. We are the generation that does have eating restrictions, and many times have to take the back seat in today's world of exciting foods.

What About Leftovers?

Since most of us have only one or two people to prepare food for, judging the amount can be confusing. You had old recipes that served ten or more, and it is hard to adjust. Don't cook to have an overload of leftovers. If you shop properly, you will have less waste. All unused fruits and vegetables can be stored in a plastic bag and placed in the freezer until the next fresh soup and dessert day. Any type of food can be eaten again, just by taking the time to take it out and heat it up. Throwing it away is easier for some. Try using what you have left over before it becomes uneatable. Remember there are millions all over the world in need of nourishment.

Happy Casserole Dishes

The following casseroles are cooked on top of the stove, using the preheated oven as a warmer.

Pepper/Rice/Cheese
Yield 2-3 servings

1 cup cooked white rice

1 cup cooked brown rice

2 tbsp. margarine

1 ½cup light cottage cheese

½ cup each, red, yellow, and green bell
peppers

½ cup skim milk

1 tbsp all purpose unsalted seasoning

Clean and steam peppers with margarine, and seasoning in small non-stick skillet until vegetables are tender. Place in lightly greased casserole dish (using butter-flavored cooking spray). Combine in dish rice and cheese. Blend ingredients well. Cover and place in a warm oven until serving time.

Sweet/Sour Cream/Chicken/Cabbage
Yield 3-4 servings

12 oz. cooked chunked chicken breast

2 cup shredded red cabbage

2 cup shredded green cabbage

1 large onion

2 packages sweetener

1 cup low-fat sour cream

1 tsp. black pepper

2 cup of low sodium chicken broth

Heat skillet over medium heat. Add cabbage, chicken broth, pepper, and slice onion. Cook for 15 minutes. Drain most of the liquid from skillet Add sour cream, sweetener, and cooked chicken. Blend all ingredients together. Remove from heat. Cover until ready to serve. Place in warm oven.

Macaroni/Ham/Cheese
Yield 2-3 servings

2 cups elbow macaroni

½ cup Laughing Cow cheese

½ cup sharp chedder

1 cup low-salt diced, cooked ham

½ cup skim milk

1 tsp. black pepper

1 small red bell pepper

Cook macaroni following box directions. Eliminate the salt if called for. Drain well. In saucepan over medium heat, add milk and small thin-cut blocks of chesses. Watch and stir until most of cheese has melted. Then add black pepper, and ham still stirring. Add cheese mixture to macaroni, place in greased casserole dish.

Place in warm oven covered, until serving time. Garnish with fine fresh chopped clean red peppers.

Red bell peppers contain a large amount of antitoxins. Cow cheese is a mild spreadable cheese found in most supermarkets.

If ham is not allowed, substitute another choice of meat; just keep it right for you.

Bean/Vegetable
Yield 2-4 servings

2 cups vegetable stock

1 cup tomato sauce

1 cup baby cooked green lima beans

1 cup cooked black-eyed peas

2 tsp celery powder

1 large diced onion

½ cup fresh carrots

1 cup chopped fresh spinach

½ cup fresh button mushrooms

1 tbsp. all-purpose low-salt seasoning

1 tbsp. oregano

3 tbsp. unsalted margarine

Place in saucepan over medium heat in 2 cups vegetable stock clean cut carrots, spinach, mushrooms, onions, and dry seasonings.

When veggies are tender, drain and add to casserole dish with drained beans, melted margarine, and tomato sauce.

Blend all ingredients well. Keep covered and warm until ready to serve.

Some foods are very easy to purchase this day and time. This is what makes cooking a breeze.

Don't make cooking a problem when it can be a breeze. Stop making excuses not to cook, be good to your self.

A good choice of all purpose unsalted seasonings usually offers a good variety of different spices and herbs. This is when the practice in reading ingredients on food labels becomes a plus for you. Eat a variety of dry beans. Garbanzo (chickpeas) the calories in a ½ cup can be the high, the amount of folate (B vitamin) is also. You win some and lose some; this is why variety in eating is important.

Sweet Potato/Turkey Goodness

4 small cooked, diced sweet potatoes

2 cups well cooked diced turkey, dark meat

1 small onion (steamed)

½ cup parsley

2 tbsp. margarine

1tbsp unsalted seasoning

1 cup frozen green peas

½ tsp. cinnamon

¼ cup chicken stock

Clean and cook potatoes in 2 quarts water over high heat. When done, drain and cool. Cut in quarters. Add to unsprayed casserole dish. Combine diced turkey, steamed chopped onion, melted margarine, cinnamon, and chicken stock. Don't stir; fold all ingredients in. Cover for 5 minutes, and then add peas, lightly stirring in. Keep covered in a warm pre-heated oven until serving time. Garnish with parsley.

Remember, preheating your oven is important. Use your herbs uncooked when possible, as a garnish is perfect. Some herbs lose nutrients when cooked.

Always cook poultry done. There should be no pink fluid oozing when chicken is done.

Make The Correct Food Choices

For most of us who are restricted, it is a new step in our lives. Being able to eat what you want, and as much as you want, has been our privilege for most of our lives. Then one day you are told you have to change your way of eating; it is harmful to your health. So now the correct choices have to be made. The recipes shared in this book have been put together using all low-salt and artificial sweeteners, products low in cholesterol and saturated fats. The ending of a good meal is that it has to start good.

The food pyramid has a purpose, eat healthy. Although food is needed for the maintaining of the body, the correct amount of the proper foods has to be eaten so the ending process is healthy.

Purchase first what you should have, and then purchase what you like. Most of us as seniors do the opposite (smile). When trying new foods, herbs, and spices, take it slow. Restrictions in condiments are not easy. They bring so much more flavor to our food.

We have cooked with pleasure, and health in mind for others for a very long time, let us cook now for our selves with the same intent in mind.

Tips For The Cook

1. Always keep your cooking area clean.
2. Don't transfer bloody materials from one place to another. Contamination is possible.
3. Familiarize yourself with the needed temperatures of the meat or meats you will be cooking; don't guess when it is done.
4. Utensils for measurements are important to use when preparing your meals. Don't guess what you need be sure.
5. Start cleaning the prep area while foods are cooking; this will give your legs less stress when the meal has been completed.
6. Cornstarch thickening is easy, thickens well, and it does not add the fat and sodium like other thickeners.
7. Seasoning, to me, is personal. In my recipes, I leave most of the seasoning to you. Low- or no-salt seasoning choices are recommended. We will never agree on seasoning; everyone's taste buds are different. I recommended Chef Paul's line of unsalted seasonings and Mrs. Dash. Both work very well for the salt-conscious cook.
8. Keep an assortment of flavorings available in your cupboard. It can be a great help in finding new tastes and savoring the old.
9. Boredom is a major obstacle when you have food restrictions. Try your best to open up to new foods.

10. Frozen vegetables can now be purchased in one serving variety packs.

11. Our kitchens can be a dangerous place if sanitation and the recognition that there is danger are ignored.

12. Keep the floors dry, and free from grease. This is something that should be done all over the home.

13. Make sure all appliances work properly at all times.

14. Don't take short cuts when it comes to appliances that carry heat, and electricity.

15. Don't get broken appliances patched up. Let them be fixed properly, or put them in the trash.

I am honored that you chose RECIPES AND MEAL PLANNING FOR H. H. S. (Happy, Healthy, Seniors) to be one of your cookbooks.

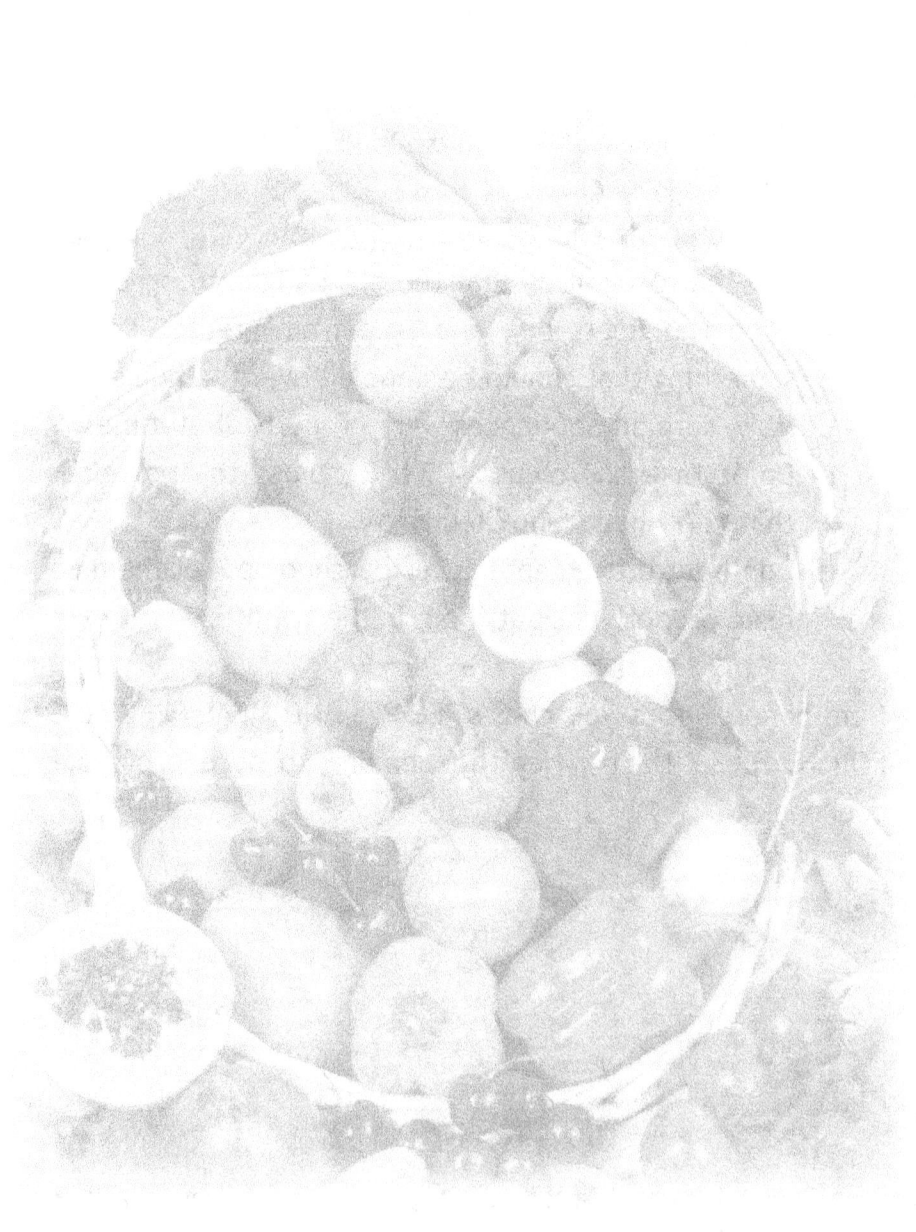

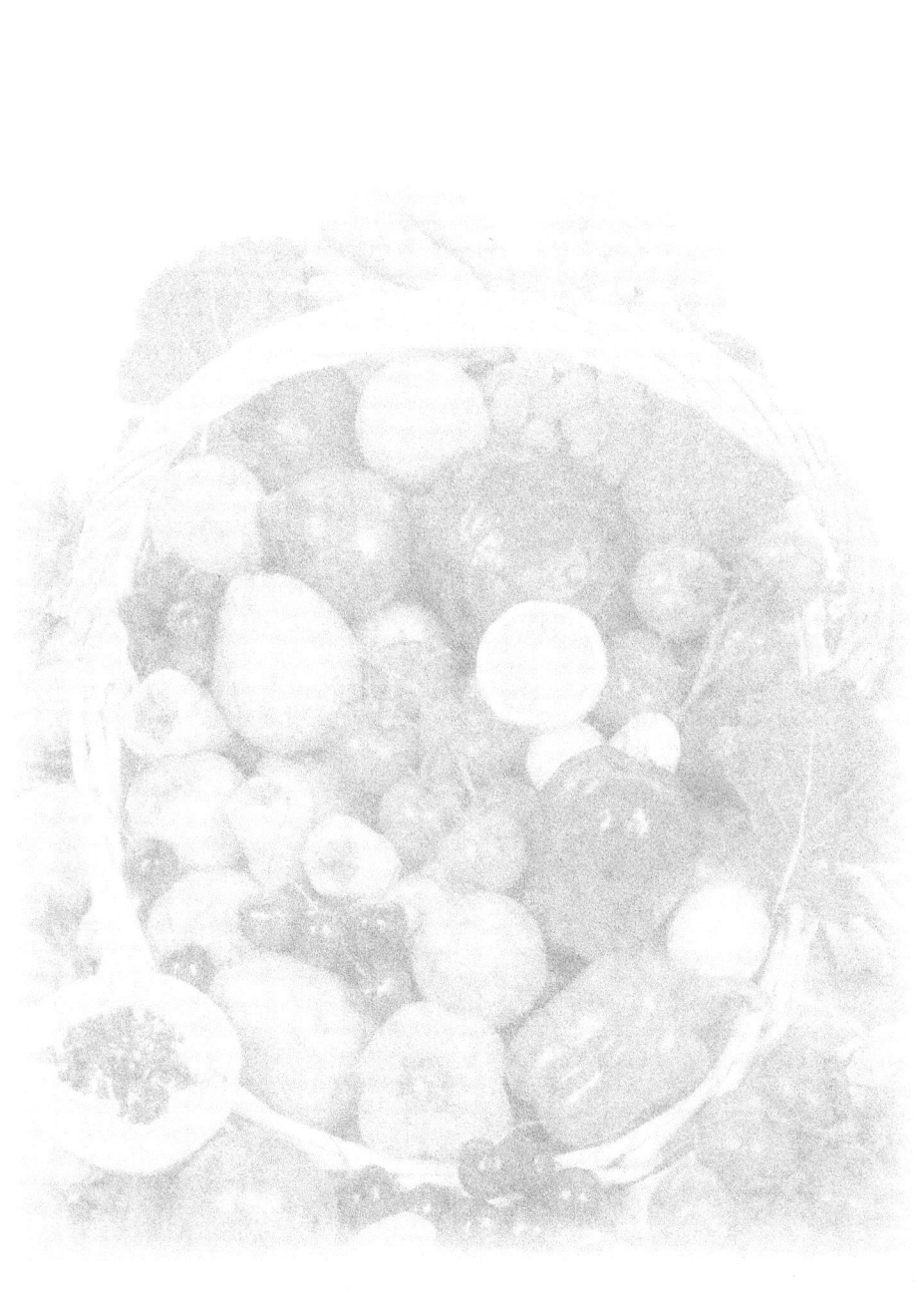

www.ingramcontent.com/pod-product-compliance
Lightning Source LLC
Chambersburg PA
CBHW060627290526
45793CB00001B/173